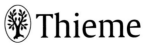

Direct Diagnosis in Radiology

Thoracic Imaging

Michael Galanski, MD
Professor
Head of Department of Radiology
Hanover Medical School
Hanover, Germany

With contributions by

Sabine Dettmer, Marc Keberle,
Jan Patrick Opherk, Kristina Ringe

285 illustrations

Thieme
Stuttgart · New York

*Library of Congress
Cataloging-in-Publication Data*
is available from the publisher.

This book is an authorized translation of the German edition published and copyrighted 2010 by Georg Thieme Verlag, Stuttgart, Germany. Title of the German edition: Pareto-Reihe Radiologie: Thorax.

Translator: John Grossman, Schrepkow, Germany

Illustrator: BITmap, Mannheim, Germany

© 2010 Georg Thieme Verlag KG
Rüdigerstrasse 14, 70469 Stuttgart, Germany
http://www.thieme.de
Thieme New York, 333 Seventh Avenue,
New York, NY 10001, USA
http://www.thieme.com

Cover design: Thieme Publishing Group
Typesetting by Ziegler + Müller,
Kirchentellinsfurt, Germany
Printed by Offizin Andersen Nexö,
Zwenkau, Germany

ISBN 978-3-13-145131-6

1 2 3 4 5 6

Important note: Medicine is an ever-changing science undergoing continual development. Research and clinical experience are continually expanding our knowledge, in particular our knowledge of proper treatment and drug therapy. Insofar as this book mentions any dosage or application, readers may rest assured that the authors, editors, and publishers have made every effort to ensure that such references are in accordance with **the state of knowledge at the time of production of the book.**

Nevertheless, this does not involve, imply, or express any guarantee or responsibility on the part of the publishers in respect to any dosage instructions and forms of applications stated in the book. **Every user is requested to examine carefully** the manufacturers' leaflets accompanying each drug and to check, if necessary in consultation with a physician or specialist, whether the dosage schedules mentioned therein or the contraindications stated by the manufacturers differ from the statements made in the present book. Such examination is particularly important with drugs that are either rarely used or have been newly released on the market. Every dosage schedule or every form of application used is entirely at the user's own risk and responsibility. The authors and publishers request every user to report to the publishers any discrepancies or inaccuracies noticed. If errors in this work are found after publication, errata will be posted at www.thieme.com on the product description page.

Michael Galanski, MD
Professor of Radiology
Head of Department of Radiology
Hanover Medical School
Hanover, Germany

Sabine Dettmer, MD
Department of Radiology
Hanover Medical School
Hanover, Germany

Marc Keberle, MD
Brüderkrankenhaus St. Josef
Municipal Hospital
Department of Diagnostic Radiology
and Nuclear Medicine
Paderborn, Germany

Jan Patrick Opherk, MD
Department of Radiology
Hanover Medical School
Hanover, Germany

Kristina Imeen Ringe, MD
Department of Radiology
Hanover Medical School
Hanover, Germany

Contents

Contents

ACTH	Adrenocorticotropic hormone	**ERS**	European Respiratory Society
AFP	Alpha-fetoprotein	**FDG**	Fluoro-18-deoxyglucose
ANCA	Antineutrophilic cytoplasmic antibodies	FEV_1	Forced expiratory volume in 1 second
ARDS	Acute respiratory distress syndrome	**FEV25–75%**	Forced expiratory volume in mid-expiratory phase
ATS	American Thoracic Society	**HCG**	Human chorionic gonadotrophin
AVM	Arteriovenous malformation	**HIV**	Human immuno-deficiency virus
CAD	Computer-aided detection	**HU**	Hounsfield units
CNS	Central nervous system	**HRCT**	High-resolution CT
COPD	Chronic obstructive pulmonary disease	**MALT**	Mucosal associated lymphoid tissue
CSF	Cerebrospinal fluid	**MIBG**	123I-metaiodoben-zylguanidine
CT	Computed tomography	**MIP**	Maximum intensity projection
CTA	CT angiography	**MRI**	Magnetic resonance imaging
DOTATOC-PET	Gadolinium-dodecyl tetra acetic acid-D-phenyl(1)-tyrosine (3)-octreotide positron emission tomography	**PEEP**	Positive end-expiratory pressure
		PET	Positron emission tomography
DSA	Digital subtraction angiography	**TNF**	Tumor necrosis factor

Definition

Abnormal communication between a pulmonary artery or arteriole and a pulmonary vein or venule.

▶ **Epidemiology**
Rare • 80–90% occur in the setting of hereditary hemorrhagic telangiectasia (Osler–Weber–Rendu disease).

▶ **Etiology, pathophysiology, pathogenesis**
Usually congenital, rarely acquired (traumatic) • Sporadic, usually solitary • Osler–Weber–Rendu disease usually involves multiple lesions • An arterial feeder and draining vein are usually present.

Imaging Signs

▶ **Modality of choice**
CT, CTA.

▶ **Radiographic findings**
Round or lobulated opacity surrounded by normal-appearing tissue; lesions with larger caliber feeding and draining vessels typically have a vascular pedicle extending toward the hilum.

▶ **CT findings**
Findings are similar to radiography and include a round or lobulated lesion • The vascular relationship is often demonstrated only on cine mode, in which the diagnosis can be made by interactive observation • Plain scans show density values typical of vascular structures • Enhancement typical of vascular structures occurs after contrast administration.

▶ **Pathognomonic findings**
Round or lobulated lesion with a vascular pedicle.

Clinical Aspects

▶ **Typical presentation**
Usually the lesion is an asymptomatic incidental finding; hypoxemia and signs of heart failure occur only with a high shunt volume • One-third of patients have a history of transient ischemic attack or stroke (venous thrombi) or cerebral abscesses (bypassing of the pulmonary capillary filter).

▶ **Therapeutic options**
Balloon embolization, coiling, or resection.

▶ **Course and prognosis**
In Osler–Weber–Rendu disease the course and prognosis depend on the underlying disorder.

▶ **What does the clinician want to know?**
Diagnosis • Location • In Osler–Weber–Rendu disease it may be advisable to obtain CT scans of carriers in the family for early detection of pulmonary arteriovenous malformation.

Fig. 1.1 AVM in Osler–Weber–Rendu disease. CT (MIP) shows multilocular tortuous and expanded vascular structures with shunt connections in the periphery that were not visualized on the chest radiograph to this degree of detail.

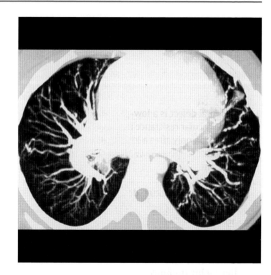

Differential Diagnosis

Pulmonary nodule	– Does not show enhancement typical of vascular structures
	– Feeding vessels are not functionally expanded in contrast to AVM

Tips and Pitfalls

Can be misinterpreted as a pulmonary nodule or suspected malignancy.

Selected References

Langer R, Langer M. Value of CT in the diagnosis of pulmonary arteriovenous shunts. Cardiovasc Intervent Radiol 1984; 7: 277–279

White RI et al. Pulmonary arteriovenous malformations: diagnosis and transcatheter embolotherapy. J Vasc Interv Radiol 1996; 7: 787–804

Definition

▶ **Epidemiology**
Most common causes include defect with left-to-right shunt, atrial septal defect, ventricular septal defect, and patent ductus arteriosus.

▶ **Etiology, pathophysiology, pathogenesis**
Left-to-right shunt increases the volume of blood in the pulmonary circulation • Atrial septal defect is a low-pressure shunt with volume overload; it leads to increased vascular resistance in the pulmonary circulation with pulmonary arterial hypertension only after a long time • Ventricular septal defect is a high-pressure shunt with rapidly increasing vascular resistance and pulmonary arterial hypertension; shunt flow reverses when pressure is equalized (Eisenmenger reaction) • Patent ductus arteriosus is a high-pressure shunt with hemodynamic effects similar to ventricular septum defect.

Imaging Signs

▶ **Modality of choice**
Echocardiography, MRI.

▶ **Radiographic findings**
Findings are positive only where shunt volume exceeds 40%; the findings then include a prominent pulmonary artery segment as well as prominent lung arteries with a slender aorta • Pulmonary vascular structures are enlarged • Normal or slightly widened heart silhouette • Abrupt changes in vascular caliber and signs of right heart strain only occur with pulmonary arterial hypertension • Ventricular septal defect and patent ductus arteriosus are associated with enlargement of the left atrium, and patent ductus arteriosus with a dilated ascending aorta.

▶ **MRI findings**
Visualizes shunt location and morphology • Allows estimation of shunt volume (quantification of blood flow in the ascending aorta and pulmonary trunk).

▶ **Pathognomonic findings**
Prominent central and peripheral vascular structures.

Clinical Aspects

▶ **Typical presentation**
Shunts with minimal hemodynamic effects are often asymptomatic or minimally symptomatic • Clinically relevant shunts lead to right heart failure in atrial septal defect and left heart failure in ventricular septal defect.

▶ **Therapeutic options**
Early correction.

▶ **Course and prognosis**
Prognosis is good with early correction • Unfavorable with pulmonary arterial hypertension and Eisenmenger reaction.

Fig. 1.2 Atrial septal defect (ostium secundum) with a 60% left-to-right shunt in a 41-year-old woman. The plain chest radiographs show a widened heart silhouette with signs of right heart strain (prominent pulmonary trunk and broad area of contact between the anterior wall of the heart and the sternum) and a conspicuously narrow aorta. In contrast, the hila are prominent with increased pulmonary vasculature without signs of redistribution.

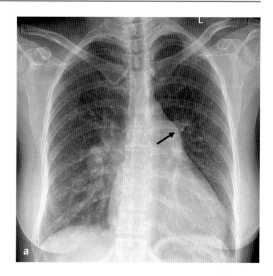

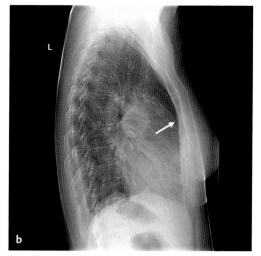

▶ **What does the clinician want to know?**
Shunt location and morphology ● Shunt volume ● Valvular and ventricular function ● Signs of heart failure.

Differential Diagnosis

Increased cardiac output   – Hyperthyroidism
– Polycythemia
– Hypervolemia

Tips and Pitfalls

Defects with "small" shunt volume (< 50%) are not detectable on plain radiographs.

Selected References

Baron MG, Book WM. Congenital heart disease in the adult. Radiol Clin North Am 2004; 42: 675–690

Steiner RM, et al. Congenital heart disease in the adult patient: The value of plain film chest radiology. J Thorac Imaging 1995; 10: 1–25

Wang ZJ et al. Cardiovascular shunts: MR imaging evaluation. Radiographics 2003; 23: 181–194

Definition

Anomalous, vertically coursing right pulmonary vein, often associated with other congenital malformations: Pulmonary venolobar syndrome • Congenital hypoplastic lung • Pulmonary hypoplasia with atypical pulmonary venous drainage • Pulmonary sequestration.

▶ **Epidemiology**
  Rare ($2:100\,000$).

▶ **Etiology, pathophysiology, pathogenesis**
  Congenital malformation in which the right or, rarely, the left pulmonary vein drains directly into a systemic vein (usually the subphrenic inferior vena cava, less often the hepatic vein or portal vein), the right atrium, or the coronary sinus; this may lead to a left-to-right shunt and pulmonary hypertension. A septal defect is present in 25% of all cases • In congenital hypogenetic lung there is malformation of the right lung with stunted development of the bronchovascular system; the lung may be supplied by a systemic artery.

Imaging Signs

▶ **Modality of choice**
  MRA or CT is preferable to plain radiography.

▶ **Radiographic findings**
  Anomalous right pulmonary vein travels vertically and then curves medially at the level of the diaphragm like a scimitar • The stunted right lung may show associated anomalies such as prominent bronchovascular structures, a high-riding diaphragm, and mediastinal shift toward the affected side.

▶ **CT findings**
  Precisely visualizes pulmonary venous drainage and systemic arterial supply • Modality of choice for demonstrating associated malformations such as pulmonary hypoplasia, horseshoe lung, tracheal diverticulum, bronchiectasis, cardiac anomalies (usually septal defects), and supply from a systemic artery.

▶ **MRA findings**
  Findings are similar to CT.

▶ **Angiography**
  No longer indicated as a primary diagnostic modality • CTA and MRA have largely replaced conventional angiography.

▶ **Pathognomonic findings**
  Anomalous vertically coursing right pulmonary vein.

Clinical Aspects

▶ **Typical presentation**
  Half of all cases are asymptomatic • Recurrent pulmonary infections • Signs of a left-to-right shunt (dyspnea during physical exertion).

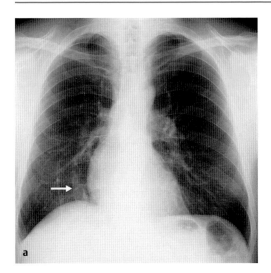

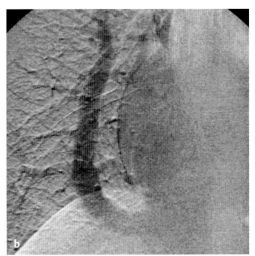

Fig. 1.3 Scimitar syndrome.

a The plain chest radiograph shows a prominent anomalous pulmonary vein traveling parallel to the right wall of the heart and disappearing in the right cardiophrenic angle (arrow).

b The vein drains into the inferior vena cava. (Digital subtraction angiography [DSA].)

▶ **Therapeutic options**
No specific therapy is required ● Surgical correction of associated cardiac anomalies or management of bronchiectasis may be indicated.

▶ **Course and prognosis**
Patients with an isolated anomalous pulmonary venous connection have normal life expectancy ● Otherwise dependant on associated cardiovascular anomalies.

▶ **What does the clinician want to know?**
Identify other developmental anomalies ● Quantification of shunt ● Signs of pulmonary arterial hypertension.

Differential Diagnosis

Platelike atelectasis	– Usually horizontal or coursing laterally and slightly cranially
Pulmonary sequestration	– Shadow in the paravertebral costophrenic angle, more common on the left than on the right – No atypical pulmonary vein
MacLeod/Swyer–James syndrome	– Obstructive emphysema secondary to bronchiolitis obliterans – Normal pulmonary venous drainage
Atypical "wandering" pulmonary vein	– Atypical course of pulmonary vein with normal drainage into the left atrium

Tips and Pitfalls

Findings can be very subtle ● Look for a vessel with an atypical course in any small right lung with increased transparency.

Selected References

Cirillo RL. The Scimitar sign. Radiology 1998; 206: 623–624

Woodring JH, Howard TA, Kanga JF. Congenital pulmonary venolobar syndrome. Radiographics 1994; 14: 349–369

Zylak CJ et al. Developmental anomalies in the adult: radiographic–pathologic correlation. Radiographics 2002; 22: 25–43

Definition

Pulmonary tissue with systemic arterial supply that has no connection with the normal tracheobronchial system.

▶ **Epidemiology**

Accounts for 0.15–6.4% of congenital pulmonary malformations • Manifests in childhood.

▶ **Etiology, pathophysiology, pathogenesis**

Congenital foregut malformation • More common on the left side than the right • There are several types: Intralobar sequestrations (75–80% of all cases) occur within the pleura of the normal lung • Extralobar sequestrations form an accessory lobe outside the normal pleura • An accessory lung is a bronchopulmonary sequestration with a rudimentary bronchus.

Imaging Signs

▶ **Modality of choice**

CT, CTA.

▶ **Radiographs**

Smoothly demarcated oval or triangular shadow in the left posteromedial basal region • Perforation leads to development of multilocular fluid-filled or air-filled cysts • Two-thirds of these anomalies occur in the left lung in the posterior segment of the lower lobe.

▶ **CT and MRI findings**

Smoothly demarcated oval or triangular shadow in a typical location • Cysts following perforation • CTA demonstrates systemic arterial supply from the aorta • Hyperinflation due to air trapping (intralobar pulmonary sequestration).

▶ **Angiographic findings**

Supplied by the thoracic aorta (70% of all cases), abdominal aorta (20%), or an intercostal artery (5%) • Drained by pulmonary veins (intralobar sequestration), systemic veins, or the portal vein (extralobar sequestration).

▶ **Pathognomonic findings**

Oval or triangular shadow (with or without cystic components) in a typical location (the medioposterior basal segment of the left lung) with systemic arterial supply.

Clinical Aspects

▶ **Typical presentation**

Extralobar sequestration is usually asymptomatic • A pulmonary infection is usually the initial finding in intralobar pulmonary sequestration • Recurrent pneumonia • Superinfection • Hemoptysis.

▶ **Therapeutic options**

Resection • Embolization.

Fig. 1.4 Pulmonary sequestration as an incidental finding in a 68-year-old man.

a The plain chest radiograph shows a circumscribed convex shadow in the right cardiophrenic angle.

b CT (oblique coronal MIP) visualizes the finding as a sharply demarcated, faintly lobular intrapulmonary consolidation communicating with the descending thoracic aorta.

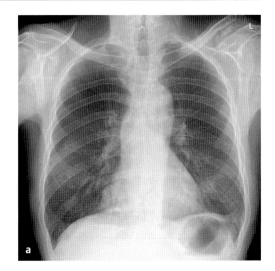

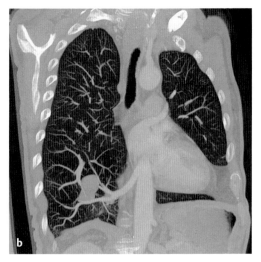

▶ **Course and prognosis**
Prognosis after resection is good • Untreated cases can develop superinfection, enteropulmonary fistulas, or hemorrhages (intracystic bleeding, hemothorax) • Extralobar sequestration is often associated with other developmental anomalies.

▶ **What does the clinician want to know?**
Confirm the tentative diagnosis by demonstrating systemic arterial supply.

Differential Diagnosis

Pneumonia	– Remission with treatment
Atelectasis	– Remission with treatment
Tumor in the paravertebral posterior lower mediastinum	– Neuroblastoma in children: calcifications, metabolites in the urine (vanillylmandelic acid) – Other neurogenic tumor: skeletal involvement

Tips and Pitfalls

Can be misinterpreted in radiographs as bronchopneumonic infiltrate.

Selected References

Franco J et al. Diagnosis of pulmonary sequestration by spiral CT angiography. Thorax 1998; 53: 1088–1092

Frazier AA et al. Intralobar sequestration: Radiologic–pathologic correlation. Radiographics 1997; 17: 725–745

Shanmugam G. Adult congenital lung disease. Eur J Cardiothorac Surg 2005; 28: 483–489

Definition

▶ **Epidemiology**
Unilateral atresia of the pulmonary artery ● Rare.

▶ **Etiology, pathophysiology, pathogenesis**
Developmental anomaly ● Twice as common on the left than on the right ● Usually associated with a right aortic arch ● Often occurs in association with other cardiac anomalies (septal defect, coarctation of the aorta, patent ductus arteriosus).

Imaging Signs

▶ **Modality of choice**
CT, MRI.

▶ **Radiographic findings**
Small ipsilateral hemithorax with hypoplastic hilum and faint vascular structures (irregular due to collaterals) ● Contralateral hypertransradiant hemithorax with prominent vascular structures ● Mediastinal shift toward the affected side ● Right aortic arch.

▶ **CT and MRI findings**
Unilateral absence of the pulmonary artery with hypoplastic, irregular pulmonary arterial architecture, because of collateral supply via the bronchial, intercostal, and other adjacent arteries.

▶ **Pathognomonic findings**
Small left hemithorax with apparently absent hilum and contralateral aortic arch.

Clinical Aspects

▶ **Typical presentation**
Recurrent infections ● Dyspnea ● Hemoptysis ● Occurs in adolescents and young adults ● Asymptomatic in about 15% of all cases ● Possible complications include pulmonary arterial hypertension in pregnancy and edema at high altitude.

▶ **Therapeutic options**
None ● Hemoptysis may require embolization or pneumonectomy.

▶ **Course and prognosis**
Depend on associated cardiac disorders.

▶ **What does the clinician want to know?**
Determine the cause and specifically exclude a tumor.

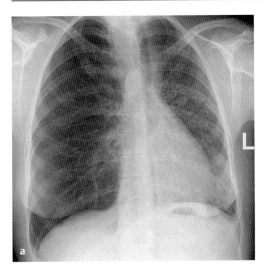

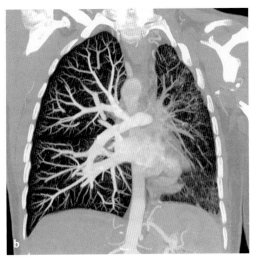

Fig. 1.5 Pulmonary artery atresia in a 45-year-old woman.

a The plain chest radiograph shows a small left hemithorax with leftward shift of the mediastinum and right aortic arch. The vascular structures over the left lung appear irregular.

b CT demonstrates atresia of the left pulmonary artery with altered parenchymal texture with irregular, slightly more pronounced yet fine vascular architecture with collaterals.

Differential Diagnosis

MacLeod/Swyer–James syndrome	– CT shows a mixed picture with hyperinflated and normally inflated areas – Bronchiectatic tissue remodeling with thickened bronchi in collapsed, scarred lung segments
Central bronchial carcinoma	– Tumor ventilation defect with perfusion defect from reflex vasoconstriction – Paradoxical hilus sign – Intact pulmonary artery
Foreign body aspiration	– Ventilation defect (atelectasis) from foreign-body aspiration with perfusion defect from reflex vasoconstriction – History – Intact pulmonary artery

Tips and Pitfalls

Can be misinterpreted in radiographs as tumor-related pathology or as MacLeod/ Swyer–James syndrome.

Selected References

Ten Harkel AD, Blom NA, Ottenkamp J. Isolated unilateral absence of a pulmonary artery: case report and review of the literature. Chest 2002; 122: 1471–1477

Definition

▶ **Epidemiology**
Very rare • Bronchus terminates in a blind pouch that does not communicate with the central bronchial system.

▶ **Etiology, pathophysiology, pathogenesis**
Results from a primary developmental anomaly with defective branching of the bronchial system or secondary circumscribed local necrosis • Most common location is the left upper lobe (two-thirds of cases).

Imaging Signs

▶ **Modality of choice**
CT.

▶ **Radiographic findings**
Typical triad of findings: A sharply demarcated focal opacity close to the hilum (mucus plug in the proximal atretic bronchus); local emphysema in the dependent segment from collateral air drift; and reduced vascularity in the dependent segment.

▶ **CT findings**
Similar to radiography; a "truncated" bronchus is directly visualized in a segment ventilated by collateral air drift.

▶ **Pathognomonic findings**
Characteristic triad (see "Radiographic findings").

Clinical Aspects

▶ **Typical presentation**
The condition is an asymptomatic, incidental finding in most cases • Less often patients present with dyspnea, asthmatic complaints, or recurrent infection.

▶ **Therapeutic options**
Usually no treatment is required.

▶ **Course and prognosis**
Good.

▶ **What does the clinician want to know?**
Evaluate the abnormal incidental finding • Exclude a tumor • Exclude other possible causes of local hyperinflation.

Differential Diagnosis

Congenital lobar emphysema	– Occurs in infants – Usually there is massive hyperinflation of the upper lobe with mediastinal shift and compressive atelectasis of adjacent ipsilateral lung segments
Bronchial obstruction with valve mechanism	– Obstructive extraluminal or intraluminal pathology leading to hyperinflation

Fig. 1.6 Bronchial atresia in the right lower lobe in a 20-year-old man.

a Localized emphysema of the right lower lobe was an incidental finding on the plain chest radiograph (CT scan).

b The radiographic finding correlates on CT with significant hyperinflation and increased transradiancy accompanied by reduced vascularity. The vessels are reduced in caliber and show straighter courses. In the center of this area there is an ectatic bronchus terminating in a blind pouch, without mucus retention (arrow).

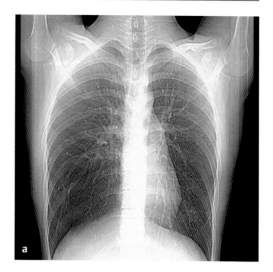

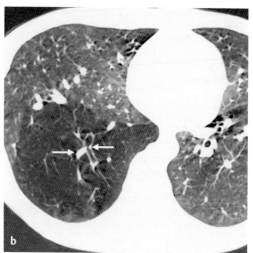

Tips and Pitfalls

Can be misinterpreted as a tumor with poststenotic hyperinflation.

Selected References

Matsushima H et al. Congenital bronchial atresia: radiologic findings in 9 patients. JCAT 2002; 26: 860–864

Murat A et al. Bronchial atresia of the right lower lobe. Acta Radiol 2005; 46: 480–483

Disorders of the Airways

Definition

Increase in transradiancy of a lung field.

▶ **Etiology, pathophysiology, pathogenesis**
One of several causes may be involved: Primary congenital pulmonary artery hypoplasia • MacLeod/Swyer-James syndrome, i.e., hypoplasia of pulmonary parenchyma including the territory of the pulmonary artery secondary to viral infection in the first 8 years of life prior to complete maturation of the lung • Perfusion defect from reflex vasoconstriction where a central bronchial obstruction (central bronchial carcinoma, bronchial adenoma, or endobronchial foreign body) creates a ventilation defect.

Imaging Signs

▶ **Modality of choice**
CT.

▶ **Radiographic findings**
Hypertransradiant hemithorax with hypoperfusion • Signs of hyperinflation in the presence of a central bronchial obstruction.

▶ **CT findings**
Depend on the cause • *Pulmonary artery hypoplasia:* Hypoplastic pulmonary arterial system with otherwise normal parenchymal texture • *MacLeod/Swyer–James syndrome:* Mixed picture with hyperinflated and normally inflated areas, bronchiectatic tissue remodeling with thickened bronchi in collapsed, scarred lung segments • Central bronchial carcinoma with bronchial and/or pulmonary artery obstruction • Endobronchial obstruction due to tumor or foreign body.

▶ **Pathognomonic findings**
Depend on the cause.

Clinical Aspects

▶ **Typical presentation**
Asymptomatic incidental finding in MacLeod/Swyer–James syndrome and in pulmonary artery hypoplasia • Symptomatic in tumor cases.

▶ **Therapeutic options**
Depend on the cause and/or underlying disorder.

▶ **Course and prognosis**
Depend on the cause and/or underlying disorder.

▶ **What does the clinician want to know?**
Determine the cause and specifically exclude a tumor.

Differential Diagnosis

MacLeod/Swyer–James syndrome	– CT shows a mixed picture with hyperinflated and normally inflated areas – Bronchiectatic tissue remodeling with thickened bronchi in collapsed, scarred lung segments
Pulmonary artery hypoplasia	– More common on the left than right; hypoplastic pulmonary artery system – Hemithorax smaller on the affected side – No air trapping
Central bronchial carcinoma	– Tumor ventilation defect with perfusion defect from reflex vasoconstriction – Paradoxical hilus sign
Endobronchial tumor (bronchial adenoma)	– Tumor ventilation defect with perfusion defect from reflex vasoconstriction – Hyperinflation with valve mechanism; CT shows endobronchial mass blocking the lumen
Foreign body aspiration	– Ventilation defect from foreign-body aspiration with perfusion defect from reflex vasoconstriction – Hyperinflation with valve mechanism – Air trapping – History; CT shows endobronchial foreign body

Tips and Pitfalls

Can be confused with off-center grid, post-mastectomy, and unilateral atrophy of the pectoralis muscles.

Selected References

Lucaya J et al. Spectrum of manifestations of Swyer-James-MacLeods syndrome. J Comput Assist Tomogr 1998; 22: 592–597

Fig. 2.1 Hypertrans-radiant hemithorax (MacLeod/Swyer–James syndrome) in an 18-year-old woman. The plain chest radiograph (a) shows increased trans-radiancy of the left lung with significantly diminished vascularity. The coronal slices (**b – d**) clearly demonstrate diminished vascularity (**b**, MIP), shrinkage (**c**), and bilateral bronchiectasis (**d**).

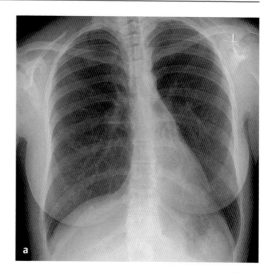

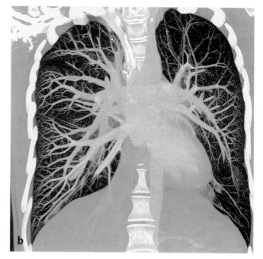

Fig. 2.1 c, d

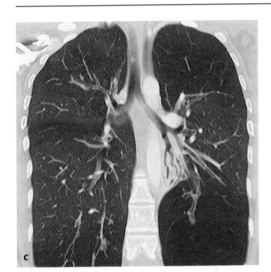

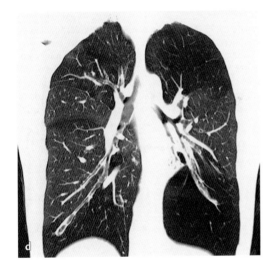

Definition

Irreversible dilation of a bronchus or bronchi, especially large and small subsegmental bronchi • Reid classification differentiates cylindrical, varicose, and cystic dilation.

▶ **Etiology, pathophysiology, pathogenesis**

Congenital (Kartagener syndrome, mucociliary dysfunction, cystic fibrosis, etc.) • Infectious (allergic bronchopulmonary aspergillosis, measles, whooping cough, tuberculosis, etc.) • Bronchial obstruction or compression (tumor, foreign body, etc.) • Pulmonary fibrosis (traction bronchiectasis) and/or thickening and inflammation of the bronchial wall • Destruction of the bronchial wall • Peribronchial fibrosis.

Imaging Signs

▶ **Modality of choice**

CT.

▶ **Radiographic findings**

Nonspecific findings • Pronounced striped pattern • Parallel stripes ("railroad track" sign) • Ring shadows.

▶ **CT findings**

"Signet ring" sign (bronchial diameter exceeds the diameter of the accompanying artery) • Bronchi fail to taper peripherally • Bronchi can be differentiated up to a subpleural depth of 1 cm • Changes in bronchial contour (cylindrical bronchi appear as tracklike parallel lines, varicose bronchi as intermittent widening of the bronchial lumina or "strings of pearls," and cystic bronchi as bunched "clusters of grapes," because of shrinkage • Nonspecific findings include bronchial thickening, fluid or mucus-filled bronchi, loss of volume, air trapping, and nodular bronchial dilation ("tree-in-bud" sign).

▶ **Pathognomonic findings**

Predilection for the posterobasal segments of the lung • "Signet ring" sign and "railroad track" sign (see above) • Ring shadow.

Clinical Aspects

▶ **Typical presentation**

Recurrent bronchopneumonia • Voluminous expectorations • Hemoptysis • Dyspnea.

▶ **Therapeutic options**

Surgery (segmental resection or lobectomy) • Pulmonary toilet • Bronchospasmolytic therapy • Specific antibiotic therapy • Active immunization against influenza and pneumococcus.

▶ **Course and prognosis**

Severity correlates with the diameter of the abnormal bronchi (cylindrical bronchiectasis has the best prognosis, cystic bronchiectasis the worst).

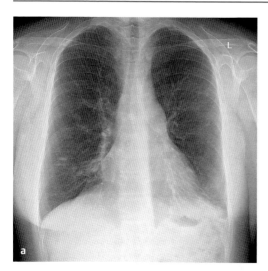

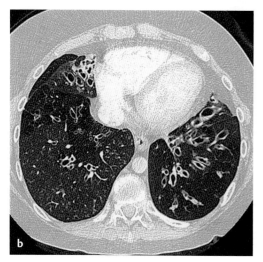

Fig. 2.2 Bronchiectasis in an 18-year-old man with immunodeficiency.

a The plain chest radiograph shows thickening of the bronchovascular bundles in the right paracardiac and left retrocardiac areas. Isolated, sharply demarcated, fine nodular densities are visible in the right lower lung field.

b On CT these changes primarily correlate with tubular bronchiectasis, occasionally concentrated, and with significant thickening of the bronchial wall and focal mucus retention.

▶ **What does the clinician want to know?**

Diagnosis of bronchiectasis • Is resection of localized bronchiectatic areas indicated? • Comorbidities detected (scarring, emphysema, abscess, empyema, broncholiths, pyemia).

Differential Diagnosis

Chronic bronchitis	– Involves the entire bronchial tree
Bronchial asthma	– No productive cough
Bullous emphysema	– No bronchial enlargement – No "signet ring" sign
Scarring and traction bronchiectasis	– Not a primary respiratory disease – Fibrotic changes in the structure of the lung

Tips and Pitfalls

Motion artefacts on the CT due to breathing can be misinterpreted as a "railroad track" sign • Reactive bronchial dilation ("reversible bronchiectasis") occurs in the presence of atelectasis.

Selected References

Cartier Y et al. Bronchiectasis: Accuracy of high resolution CT in the differentiation of specific diseases. AJR Am J Roentgenol 1999; 173: 47–52

King P, Song X, Rockwood K. Bronchiectasis. Intern Med J 2006; 36: 729–737

Definition

▶ **Epidemiology**
Inflammation of the peripheral respiratory bronchioles (diameter < 2 mm).

▶ **Etiology, pathophysiology, pathogenesis**
Acutely infectious (viruses, *Mycoplasma*, chlamydia, aspergillosis) • Chronic inflammatory (asthma, chronic bronchitis) • Panbronchiolitis • Respiratory bronchiolitis (nicotine).

Imaging Signs

▶ **Modality of choice**
CT.

▶ **Radiographic findings**
Usually normal • Reticulonodular shadowing • Pneumonic infiltrate may be present • Dystelectasis.

▶ **CT findings**
Centrilobular and peribronchovascular nodules • "Tree-in-bud" sign (usually peripheral) • Ground-glass opacities • Bronchial wall thickening • Air trapping.

▶ **Pathognomonic findings**
None • Findings such as a mosaic pattern, "tree-in-bud" sign, or centrilobular nodules are nonspecific.

Clinical Aspects

▶ **Typical presentation**
Dyspnea • Nonproductive cough (productive cough occurs in diffuse panbronchiolitis) • Fever.

▶ **Therapeutic options**
Elimination of the noxious agent • Steroids (inhalational or systemic) • Bronchoalveolar lavage.

▶ **Course and prognosis**
Prognosis is good in infections • Course is more rapid in patients with bone marrow or stem cell transplantation • In severe cases respiratory insufficiency and pulmonary fibrosis may develop • Prognosis is poor in diffuse panbronchiolitis.

Differential Diagnosis

Extrinsic allergic alveolitis or bronchiolitis	– No thickening of the bronchial wall – Rarely nicotine use
Air trapping	– Extrinsic allergic alveolitis (acute stage), no bronchial wall thickening, no nicotine use – Bronchial obstruction due to foreign body or mucus retention
Bronchiolitis obliterans with organizing pneumonia	– Nodular, usually bilateral, nonsegmental densities with air bronchogram and pleural contact

Fig. 2.3 Bronchiolitis in a 62-year-old man.

a The plain chest radiograph shows increased finely nodular shadowing, especially in the left upper field and slightly more prominent bronchial walls.

b Findings on CT are localized to the peribronchovascular region. Note the significant focal wall thickening in the small bronchi (arrowhead).

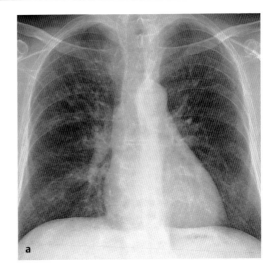

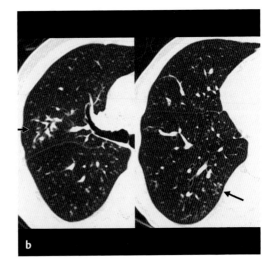

Disorders of the Airways

Tips and Pitfalls
....

False-negative diagnosis due to overlooking discrete changes.

Selected References

Hartmann TE et al. CT of bronchial and bronchiolar diseases. Radiographics 1994; 14: 991–1003

Howling SJ et al. Follicular bronchiolitis: thin-section CT and histologic findings. Radiology 1999; 212: 637–642

Müller NL, Miller RR. Diseases of the bronchioles: CT and histopathologic findings. Radiology 1995; 196: 3–12

Definition

▶ **Epidemiology**
Depends on the etiology. Every second lung transplant recipient develops a bronchiolitis obliterans syndrome within 5 years of transplantation.

▶ **Etiology, pathophysiology, pathogenesis**
Rarely idiopathic, usually secondary to infection (mycoplasmal, viral, in children especially respiratory syncytial virus), secondary to inhalation of noxious agents, as a hypersensitivity reaction (collagen diseases), secondary to transplantation (lung, heart, bone marrow), in the setting of chronic obstructive pulmonary disease • Inflammation of the respiratory bronchioles • Proliferation of submucosal and peribronchial tissue leading to concentric constriction of the respiratory bronchioles.

Imaging Signs

▶ **Modality of choice**
CT on inspiration and expiration (to detect air trapping).

▶ **Radiographic findings**
Signs of pulmonary hyperinflation of variable severity with diminished vascularity.

▶ **CT findings**
Increased transparency of the pulmonary parenchyma with narrowed vessels and signs of air trapping • On expiration the density of the affected areas fails to increase • Affected areas show increased transparency as on inspiration • Mosaic perfusion • Peribronchiolar fibrosis (rare) • In postinfectious bronchiolitis there is bronchial wall thickening and bronchiectasis • "Tree-in-bud" sign is rare.

▶ **Pathognomonic findings**
Increased transparency of the pulmonary parenchyma with narrowed vessels • Severe air trapping • Mosaic perfusion.

Clinical Aspects

▶ **Typical presentation**
Cough • Dyspnea • Fever, resembles chronic obstructive pulmonary disease but with subacute course • Primarily restrictive ventilation defect due to early complete occlusion.

▶ **Therapeutic options**
Steroids • Immunosuppression after lung transplant.

▶ **Course and prognosis**
Prognosis is good with steroid therapy.

▶ **What does the clinician want to know?**
Confirmation of tentative diagnosis in at-risk patients (post bone marrow, peripheral blood stem cell, or lung transplantation).

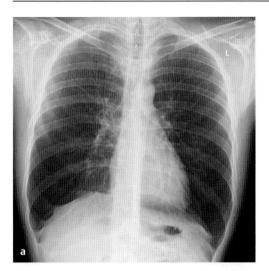

Fig. 2.4 Bronchiolitis obliterans in a 24-year-old man (graft-versus-host disease following bone marrow transplantation).

a The plain chest radiograph shows significant hyperinflation of both lungs (left more than right) with slightly more prominent bronchial walls in the perihilar region.

b CT confirms the findings and shows diminished vascularity, especially on the left side and in the right lower lobe. There was no increase in density on expiration, which is consistent with air trapping.

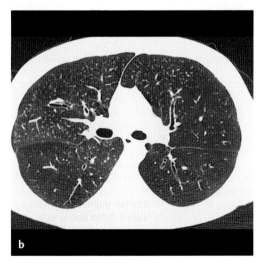

Disorders of the Airways

Differential Diagnosis

Mosaic pattern	– Constrictive bronchiolitis in graft-versus-host disease
	– Extrinsic allergic alveolitis (acute stage): no bronchial wall thickening, not associated with smoking
	– Pulmonary arterial hypertension and/or pulmonary embolism: mosaic pattern without air trapping, reduced caliber of vessels in the areas of increased transparency
	– Nodular ground-glass infiltrates in inflammatory lung disease
Air trapping	– Constrictive bronchiolitis in graft-versus-host disease
	– Extrinsic allergic alveolitis (acute stage)
	– Bronchial obstruction due to foreign body, mucus plug, or tumor
Panlobular emphysema	– Destruction of lung parenchyma
	– Predominantly in the basal lung segments
	– No mosaic perfusion
Bronchiolitis obliterans with organizing pneumonia	– Nodular, usually bilateral, nonsegmental densities with air bronchogram and pleural contact

Tips and Pitfalls

Generalized air trapping can escape detection, as can air trapping in an uncoopera-tive patient (recognizable by the absence of impression of the membranous part of the trachea).

Selected References

Bankier AA et al. Bronchiolitis obliterans syndrome in heart-lung transplant recipients: diagnosis with expiratory CT. Radiology 2001; 218: 533–539

Choi YW et al. Bronchiolitis obliterans syndrome in lung transplant recipients: correlation of CT findings with bronchiolitis obliterans syndrome stage. J Thorac Imaging 2003; 18: 72–79

Hansell DM et al. Obliterative bronchiolitis: individual CT signs of small airway disease and functional correlation. Radiology 1997; 203: 721–726

Definition

Pulmonary disorder characterized by increased resistance to airflow • FEV_1/FVC < 70%.

▶ **Epidemiology**

Among smokers 15–20% develop COPD.

▶ **Etiology, pathophysiology, pathogenesis**

Inflammatory reaction of the large and small airways caused by inhaled noxious agents and involving bronchial obstruction, mucociliary dysfunction, and structural changes (destruction) • Disruption of the physiologic balance between proteases and protease inhibitors • Oxidative stress.

Imaging Signs

▶ **Modality of choice**

CT.

▶ **Radiographic findings**

Often normal • Bronchial walls may appear more pronounced ("tramline" shadows) • Signs of right heart strain.

▶ **CT findings**

Thickened bronchial walls • Mucus retention • Centrilobular emphysema may be present • Enlarged central pulmonary arteries.

▶ **Pathognomonic findings**

Chronic bronchitis and COPD are not radiologic diagnoses • Morphologic findings on the radiograph essentially depend on the severity of the disorder.

Clinical Aspects

▶ **Typical presentation**

Productive cough • Dyspnea • Hemoptysis • Clubbed fingers.

Reduced FEV_1, abnormal blood gases, elevated C-reactive protein.

Functional grading FEV_1 (GOLD): Stages 0–IV (I: mild, ≥ 80%; II: moderate, 50–79%; III: severe, 30–49%; IV: very severe, < 30%).

Systemic components of COPD: weight loss, cachexia ("pink puffer" • pulmonary cachexia in COPD with emphysema) • osteoporosis, muscle atrophy • heart failure, atherosclerosis.

▶ **Therapeutic options**

Tobacco abstinence • Bronchodilators • Inhalational corticosteroids • Oxygen therapy.

▶ **Course and prognosis**

Chronic progressive disorder • Mortality depends on the stage.

▶ **What does the clinician want to know?**

The diagnosis is based on clinical and especially functional parameters • Radiology plays a supporting role by determining the extent of emphysema and identifying complications.

Fig. 2.5   COPD in a 48-year-old woman smoker. Morphologic findings on the radiograph are hardly impressive except in advanced cases with recurrent infection. The plain chest radiograph shows a low-lying, flattened diaphragm consistent with hyperinflation and a slightly increased bronchovascular shadowing in the basal lung segments. Vascularity is minimal in the upper fields due to emphysematous changes.

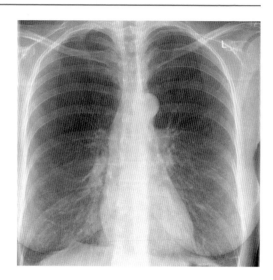

Differential Diagnosis

Asthma	– Hyperinflation without parenchymal destruction
Emphysema	– Centrilobular emphysema is often a component of COPD
Bronchiectasis	– Frequent complication of chronic bronchitis

Selected References

Takasugi JE, Godwin JD. Radiology of chronic obstructive pulmonary disease. Radiol Clin North Am 1998; 36: 29–55

Vogelmeier C et al. [Pathogenese der COPD.] Internist 2006; 47: 885–894 [In German]

Definition

Metabolic disorder of exocrine glands with abnormal mucus secretion.

▶ **Epidemiology**
Most common congenital metabolic disorder in Caucasians.

▶ **Etiology, pathophysiology, pathogenesis**
Autosomal recessive genetic defect • Defective chloride transport causes exocrine glands to excrete highly viscous mucus • Compromised mucociliary clearance • Recurrent bronchopulmonary infections.

Imaging Signs

▶ **Modality of choice**
Radiographs, CT.

▶ **Radiographic findings**
Hyperinflation • Bronchial wall thickening • Bronchiectasis with mucus retention • Atelectasis • Cysts • Pneumothorax • Hilar lymphadenopathy.

▶ **CT findings**
Bronchial wall thickening, especially in the central and upper lobes • Cystic-varicose bronchiectasis, more often in the upper lobes than lower lobes • Mucus retention • "Tree-in-bud" sign • Mosaic perfusion • Air trapping.

▶ **Pathognomonic findings**
Severe cystic-varicose bronchiectasis, primarily in the upper lobes • Manifestations in other organ systems (meconium ileus, pancreatic exocrine insufficiency).

Clinical Aspects

▶ **Typical presentation**
Usually manifests itself in infancy • Chronic recurrent bronchopulmonary infections (especially *Pseudomonas, Aspergillus,* and mycobacteria) • Hemoptysis • Pneumothorax.

▶ **Therapeutic options**
Mucolytic therapy (postural drainage, percussion) • Medical therapy (specific antibiotic therapy, bronchodilators, pancreatic enzymes) • Lung transplant • Somatic gene therapy (transfer of healthy *CFTR* genes).

▶ **Course and prognosis**
Shorter life expectancy (course is often milder where initial manifestation occurs in adulthood) • Pulmonary hypertension and respiratory insufficiency occur over time • Pancreatic exocrine insufficiency.

▶ **What does the clinician want to know?**
Evaluation of the clinical course using semiquantitative scoring systems such as the Crispin–Norman score in children • Extent of changes, especially bronchiectasis on CT.

Fig. 2.6   Cystic fibrosis in a 34-year-old woman. In addition to slight pulmonary hyperinflation, the plain chest radiograph shows a primarily streaky pattern of increased shadowing in all lung fields, strongest in the upper and middle lung fields. The hila appear shortened and withdrawn cranially. The changes are caused by the more pronounced bronchial walls and bronchiectasis.

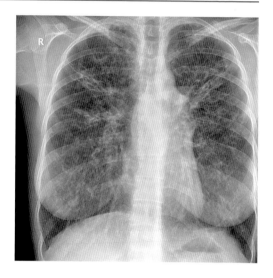

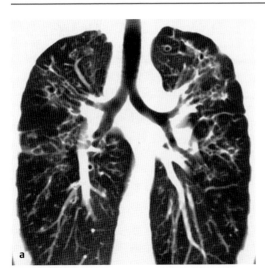

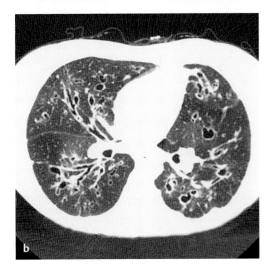

Fig. 2.7 The CT image allows better evaluation of the type and extent of the changes. The cross-sectional images reveal extensive cystic-varicose bronchiectasis.

Differential Diagnosis

Postinfectious bronchiectasis	– Usually unilateral lobar or segmental occurrence – Usually in the lower lobes
Allergic bronchopulmonary aspergillosis	– Bronchiectasis primarily in the central upper lobes – Transient infiltrates – Eosinophilia
Immotile cilia syndrome (Kartagener syndrome)	– No predilection for the upper lobe – Sinusitis – Dextrocardia

Selected References

Helbich TH et al. Cystic fibrosis: CT assessment of lung involvement in children and adults. Radiology 1999; 213: 537–544

Tiddens HA, de Jong P. Update on the implication of chest computed tomography scanning to cystic fibrosis. Curr Opin Pulm Med 2006; 12: 433–439

Wood BP. Cystic fibrosis. Radiology 1997; 204: 1–10

Definition

Permanently enlarged airspaces distal to the terminal bronchioles with destruction of the alveolar walls.

▶ **Epidemiology**

Mild forms are found in two-thirds of autopsies.

▶ **Etiology, pathophysiology, pathogenesis**

Hypoplasia secondary to bronchopulmonary disease • Atrophy, i.e., parenchymal loss occurring for example in smokers (most important etiologic factor) and patients with senile emphysema • Hyperinflation or destruction of the peripheral airways (valve mechanism, terminal-stage inflammatory disorders, alpha$_1$-antitrypsin deficiency).

Forms include: Centrilobular emphysema (smoking-related, often associated with chronic bronchitis, concomitant inflammatory changes, and fibrosis) • Panlobular emphysema (alpha$_1$-antitrypsin deficiency, MacLeod/Swyer–James syndrome, familial form) • Paraseptal emphysema.

Imaging Signs

▶ **Modality of choice**

CT.

▶ **Radiographic findings**

Sensitivity is low at about 50% (mild forms can be overlooked) • Specificity is high (> 90%) • Thoracic deformation (barrel chest deformity with increased sagittal diameter, expanded retrosternal space, wide intercostal space, blunt sinus) • Flattened, low-lying diaphragm • Diminished peripheral vascularity • Prominent hilar vessels • Hypertransparency • "Emphysema heart."

▶ **CT findings**

Demonstrates defined areas of increased transparency (emphysema threshold is < –950 HU; normal density is –750 to –900 HU).

Centrilobular emphysema involves destruction of the alveolar walls in the center of a secondary pulmonary lobule, sparing the lobular periphery and vascular structures • Predilection for cranial lung segments.

Panlobular emphysema involves destruction of the entire lobular architecture • Vascularity is diminished • Predilection for basal lung segments • A special form of this emphysema occurs in alpha$_1$-antitrypsin deficiency.

Paraseptal emphysema is bullous • Predilection for the subpleural and bronchovascular regions.

▶ **Pathognomonic findings**

The radiograph shows a typical emphysema chest with regionally or globally increased transparency and diminished peripheral vascularity • CT shows destruction of the alveolar walls.

Fig. 2.8 Pulmonary emphysema in a 50-year-old man. The plain chest radiograph shows a bell-shaped chest with a low-lying flattened diaphragm. Findings include consistently diminished vascularity in the lung fields. Individual vessels appear slightly bowed. Slender, oscillating heart shadow with a prominent pulmonary segment.

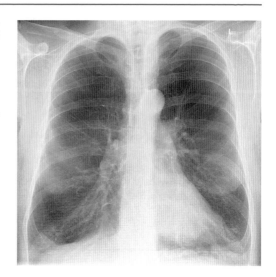

Clinical Aspects

▶ **Typical presentation**

The extent of dysfunction depends primarily on the severity of the emphysema and less on the type ● Senile and hyperinflation emphysema are often asymptomatic ● The "pink puffer" is a dyspneic pulmonary patient with dyspnea on exercise, nonproductive cough, and relatively normal blood gas levels ● The "blue bloater" is a patient with normal breathing but bronchial problems, who has cyanosis and chronic recurrent bronchitis ● Signs of pulmonary hypertension ● Lung volume and residual volume are increased; FEV_1 and diffusion capacity are reduced.

▶ **Therapeutic options**

Tobacco abstinence ● Infection prophylaxis ● Medical therapy (bronchodilators, $alpha_1$-antitrypsin substitution) ● Respiratory therapy ● Surgery (reduction of lung volume, bullectomy, lung transplant).

▶ **Course and prognosis**

Complications include spontaneous pneumothorax and recurrent bronchopulmonary infections ● Limitation of lung function correlates with the extent of parenchymal changes ● Prognosis is poor in advanced-stage disease.

▶ **What does the clinician want to know?**

Extent of parenchymal destruction ● Differentiate localized emphysema from generalized emphysema.

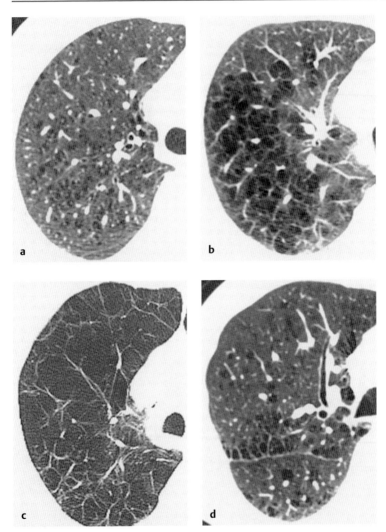

Fig. 2.9 Quantification and classification of emphysema requires CT. Centrilobular emphysema (**a**) is characterized by finely nodular radiolucencies consistent with hyperinflated alveoli in the center of the acini. Panlobular emphysema (**c**) is characterized by generalized hyperinflation with parenchymal destruction. Transitional forms (**b**) with areas of centrilobular and panlobular emphysema are common. Paraseptal emphysema is a common finding and usually not clinically significant (**d**). Here it occurs in combination with centrilobular emphysema.

Differential Diagnosis

Pulmonary cyst, cystic lesions	– Visible wall structures
Bronchial asthma	– No parenchymal destruction – Hyperinflation may be reversible after administering bronchodilators
Bronchiolitis obliterans	– No parenchymal destruction – Mosaic perfusion
Lymphangioleiomyomatosis	– Occurs almost exclusively in women of childbearing age – Thin-walled cysts – Chylous pleural effusion
Langerhans cell histiocytosis	– Nodular changes

Tips and Pitfalls

False-negative findings (mild emphysema can be easily overlooked on a radiograph and even on CT with wide window settings) • Extrapulmonary factors can mimic increased transparency on radiographs.

Selected References

Bankier AA, Madani A, Gevenois PA. CT quantification of pulmonary emphysema: assessment of lung structure and function. Crit Rev Comput Tomogr 2002; 43: 399–417

Foster WL et al. The emphysemas: Radiologic-pathologic correlations. Radiographics 1993; 13: 311–328

Screaton NJ, Reynolds JH. Lung volume reduction surgery for emphysema: What the radiologist needs to know. Clin Radiol 2006; 61: 237–249

Definition

Loss of volume or total collapse of part or all of a lung (referred to as lobar or segmental atelectasis depending on its extent) • Platelike or discoid atelectasis (subsegmental atelectasis) • Dystelectasis (hypoventilation).

▶ **Epidemiology**
Not a distinct disease entity per se, rather an associated condition or sequela.

▶ **Etiology, pathophysiology, pathogenesis**
Obstructive atelectasis results from bronchial occlusion and poststenotic air resorption (due to tumor, stricture, mucus plug, or foreign body) • Compressive atelectasis occurs where an intrathoracic process (pneumothorax, pleural effusion, large cysts) prevents expansion of the lung • Adhesive atelectasis occurs where the surface tension of the alveoli is so high that they collapse (as in ARDS, radiation pneumonitis) • Atelectasis can result from scarring (as in tuberculosis) • Passive atelectasis.

Imaging Signs

▶ **Modality of choice**
Radiographs. CT is used where indicated to identify the causes.

▶ **Radiographic findings**
Direct signs: Include a more or less triangular, homogeneous shadow or opacity aligned with its base toward the pleura and it apex toward the tip of the hilum.
Indirect signs: Depend on the severity of atelectasis and include volume loss and bowed fissures • Cranial shift of the diaphragm and/or mediastinal shift • Narrowed intercostal space • Compensatory hyperinflation of adjacent lung segments.
Atelectasis of the right upper lobe: Appears as an opacity in the right upper field • Apparent widening of the upper mediastinum • Trachea shifted to the right, hilum shifted cranially, upwardly bowed minor fissure (Golden's sign) • Lateral radiograph shows a triangular opacity in the anterior upper lobe.
Atelectasis of the left upper lobe: Appears as an opacity in the left upper field with an apical air crescent (the apical segment of the lower lobe) • Upper mediastinal silhouette sign • Trachea shifted to the left, hilum shifted cranially • Lateral radiograph shows an anteriorly shifted interlobar fissure coursing parallel to the anterior chest wall.
Atelectasis of the middle lobe: Appears as a wedge-like opacity with a cardiac silhouette sign • The interlobar fissures are shifted.
Atelectasis of the right or left lower lobe: Appears as a triangular opacity that partially obscures the margin of the diaphragm • The hilum is shifted caudally • The lateral radiograph shows a shift of the interlobar fissure.
Special forms: Include platelike atelectasis (segmental or subsegmental atelectasis) • Rounded atelectasis (folded lung).

▶ **CT findings**
Indirect signs are more clearly visualized • Causes are more readily identifiable; bronchial obstruction in particular is more clearly demonstrated • Contrast CT

Fig. 2.10 Atelectasis of the left lower lobe in a 38-year-old woman. Narrow wedge-shaped opacity in the left paravertebral retrocardiac area. The atelectasis has led to slightly increased transradiancy and reduced vascularity on the left side.

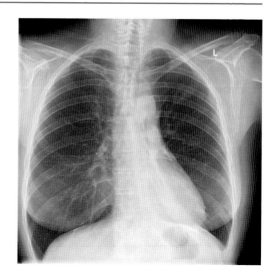

shows homogeneous enhancement (more marked and homogeneous than in a tumorous or inflammatory process).

▶ **MRI findings**
Obstructive atelectasis is hyperintense on T2-weighted images • Nonobstructive atelectasis is hypointense on T2-weighted images.

▶ **Pathognomonic findings**
Homogeneous density with signs of loss of volume in an anatomically correct location.

Clinical Aspects

▶ **Typical presentation**
Generally asymptomatic • There may be dyspnea, chest pain, cough, fever • Atelectasis of the left lower lobe occurs most often in intensive care patients.

▶ **Therapeutic options**
Atelectasis is not a distinct disease entity as such, rather an associated condition • Treatment depends on the cause and/or underlying disorder.

▶ **Course and prognosis**
Depend on the cause and/or underlying disorder.

▶ **What does the clinician want to know?**
Cause • Extent of findings.

Differential Diagnosis

Pneumonia	– Clinical aspects
	– Opacity with no volume change
	– No signs of volume loss
	– Positive air bronchogram
Pleural effusion	– Volume increase
	– Contralateral mediastinal shift
Pulmonary agenesis, pneumonectomy	– History
	– Clips and sutures
Tumor	– Often the cause of atelectasis
	– CT diagnostic studies
	– Inhomogeneous contrast enhancement
Widening of the mediastinum	– No shift of the fissures or hila

Tips and Pitfalls

Complete lobar atelectasis is easily missed ● The silhouette sign and the position of the hilum are helpful diagnostic criteria.

Selected References

Ashizawa K et al. Lobar atelectasis: diagnostic pitfalls on chest radiography. Br J Radiol 2001; 74: 89–97

Proto AV. Lobar collapse: basic concepts. Eur J Radiol 1996; 23: 9–22

Woodring JH, Reed JC. Types and mechanisms of pulmonary atelectasis. J Thorac Imaging 1996; 11: 92–108

Woodring JH, Reed JC. Radiographic manifestations of lobar atelectasis. J Thorac Imaging 1996; 11: 109–144

Definition

▶ **Epidemiology**
Sequela of inflammatory pleural reaction • Often associated with asbestos exposure.

▶ **Etiology, pathophysiology, pathogenesis**
Rounded atelectasis occurs in the setting of an atelectatic process in combination with pleuritis or a pleural effusion. The resulting scarring and adhesions prevent the collapsed segment from unfolding.

Imaging Signs

▶ **Modality of choice**
CT.

▶ **Radiographic findings**
Subpleural mass, isodense to soft tissue located in the posterior or lateral basal segment.

▶ **CT findings**
Rounded or faintly triangular, sharply demarcated mass isodense to soft tissue with broad pleural contact; vessels and bronchi converge to enter the mass in a fashion resembling the tail of a comet • There is an acute angle between mass and pleura • Typically located in the posterior or lateral basal segment • An air bronchogram is present in 60% of cases.

▶ **Pathognomonic findings**
Round subpleural mass with comet tail.

Clinical Aspects

▶ **Typical presentation**
Asymptomatic and often incidental finding in patients with a history of pleuritis or pleural effusion.

▶ **Therapeutic options**
None.

▶ **Course and prognosis**
Stationary • Lesion does not resolve spontaneously due to the pleural adhesion.

▶ **What does the clinician want to know?**
Diagnosis.

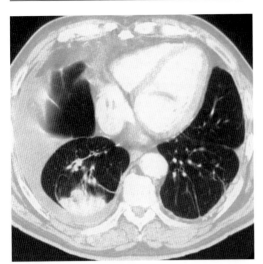

Fig. 2.11 Rounded atelectasis. The axial CT slice close to the diaphragm shows pleural adhesions and, on the right side, an encapsulated effusion with a faintly lobulated, posterior subpleural soft tissue mass. The bowed vessels converge on the mass in the fashion of a comet tail.

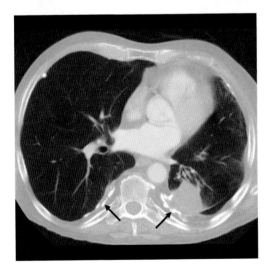

Fig. 2.12 Rounded atelectasis in calcified pleural plaques associated with asbestos exposure. Identical, nearly pathognomonic CT morphology as in Figure 2.**13**.

Differential Diagnosis

Lung carcinoma	– No comet tail
	– Symptomatic
Pleural tumor	– No comet tail
	– Obtuse angle between mass and pleura
Pulmonary infarct	– Initially triangular opacity
	– History of acute event
	– Later appears rounded ("Hampton hump")

Tips and Pitfalls

Can be misinterpreted as a tumor.

Selected References

O'Donovan P et al. Evaluation of the reliability of CT criteria in the diagnosis of round atelectasis. J Thorac Imaging 1997; 12: 54–58

Definition

Recurrent or refractory atelectasis or consolidation of the right middle lobe or the lingula segments.

▶ **Epidemiology**
Occurs in middle age • Men are affected less often than women.

▶ **Etiology, pathophysiology, pathogenesis**
The obstructive type involves bronchial obstruction from endoluminal pathology (endobronchial tumor or foreign body) or, more often, extraluminal pathology (external compression by tumor or lymph nodes) • The nonobstructive type involves bronchiectasis.

Imaging Signs

▶ **Modality of choice**
CT is preferable to plain radiography.

▶ **Radiographic findings**
Opacity with silhouette sign in the left or right paracardiac region. The opacity is projected on the silhouette of the heart on the lateral radiograph.

▶ **CT findings**
Determines whether the cause is an endoluminal mass or extraluminal compression • Associated parenchymal changes • Secondary bronchiectasis.

▶ **Pathognomonic findings**
See "Radiographic findings."

Clinical Aspects

▶ **Typical presentation**
Chronic cough.

▶ **Therapeutic options**
This depends on the cause: long-term antibiotic therapy • Tumor resection where indicated.

▶ **Course and prognosis**
This depends on the cause.

▶ **What does the clinician want to know?**
Determine the cause and exclude a tumor or foreign body • Identify chronic or irreversible changes (bronchiectasis).

Fig. 2.13 Right middle lobe syndrome in a 53-year-old woman with adenocarcinoma.

a, b The plain chest radiographs show a homogeneous opacity that correlates with the middle lobe on the lateral radiograph. The faint convexity of the minor fissure suggests a causative mass.

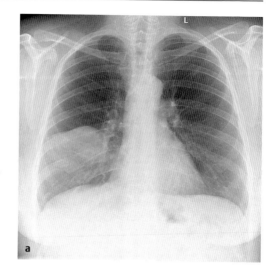

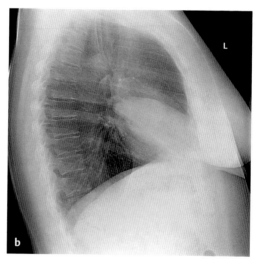

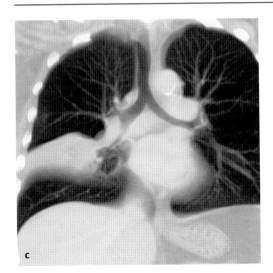

c, d The coronal and sagittal planar reformatted CT images (slab technique) confirm these findings. These images more clearly demonstrate the separation between the denser central mass and the more transparent dystelectasis.

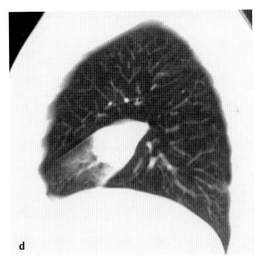

Differential Diagnosis

Middle-lobe pneumonia	– Clinical findings include symptoms of acute infection that rapidly remit under antibiotics
Atypical mycobacterial disease	– Risk patients – Chronic infiltrates
Allergic bronchopulmonary aspergillosis, cystic fibrosis	– Extensive changes not limited to the middle lobe or lingula segments
Pectus excavatum	– Pseudo-shadow (opacity) with no correlate on the lateral radiograph or CT – Depressed sternum

Tips and Pitfalls

Can be misinterpreted as pneumonia.

Selected References

Gudmundsson G, Gross TJ. Middle lobe syndrome. Am Fam Physician 1996; 53: 2547–2550
Wagner RB, Johnston MR. Middle lobe syndrome. Ann Thorac Surg 1983; 35: 679–686

Definition

Immotile cilia syndrome: Situs solitus ● Chronic sinusitis ● Bronchiectasis.
Kartagener syndrome: Situs inversus ● Chronic sinusitis ● Bronchiectasis.

▶ **Epidemiology**
Hereditary defect of ciliated cell function (1 : 2000 births) ● In about 50% of cases it is combined with situs inversus ● No sex predilection.

▶ **Etiology, pathophysiology, pathogenesis**
Abnormal bronchociliary clearance leading to recurrent bronchitis and development of bronchiectasis, showing a predilection for the middle and lower lobes.

Imaging Signs

▶ **Modality of choice**
CT is preferable to plain radiography.

▶ **Radiographic findings**
Situs inversus (50% of cases) ● More prominent bronchial walls ● Atelectasis ● Hyperinflation.

▶ **CT findings**
Bronchial wall thickening ● Bronchiectasis (middle and lower lobes) ● Bronchiolectasis ● "Tree-in-bud" sign ● Air trapping ● Segmental atelectasis or dystelectasis.

▶ **Pathognomonic findings**
Bronchiectasis (middle and lower lobes) ● Dextrocardia ● Sinusitis.

Clinical Aspects

▶ **Typical presentation**
Clinical manifestation occurs in childhood or adolescence with recurrent sinusitis, bronchitis, and pneumonia (*Haemophilus influenzae, Pseudomonas*) ● Fertility is reduced in women whereas men are sterile due to immobile spermatozoa.

▶ **Confirmation of the diagnosis**
Mucosal biopsy (nose, bronchi).

▶ **Therapeutic options**
Physical therapy ● Prophylactic mucolytics, antibiotics ● Resection of bronchiectatic segments where indicated.

▶ **Course and prognosis**
Depend on the severity and complications ● Prognosis is usually favorable with no reduction of life expectancy.

▶ **What does the clinician want to know?**
Confirmation of tentative diagnosis ● Qualitative and quantitative severity of the pulmonary changes.

Fig. 2.14   Kartagener syndrome in a 13-year-old girl.

a The plain chest radiograph shows dextrocardia with the aortic arch and azygos lobe on the right side. There is increased paracardiac and retrocardiac bronchovascular shadowing.

b On CT, this correlates with a shrunken and consolidated middle lobe with tubular bronchiectatic structures coursing through it.

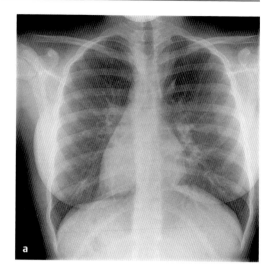

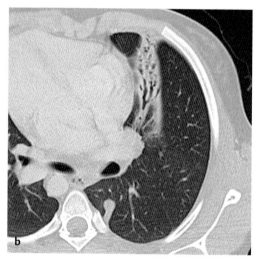

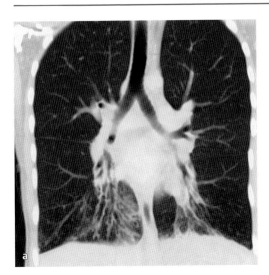

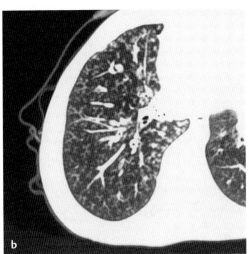

Fig. 2.15 Immotile cilia syndrome in a 15-year-old boy.

a The coronal CT image shows bilateral basal bronchiectasis and peribronchial changes with shortened bronchitic bronchi.

b Signs of hyperinflation and a severe "tree-in-bud" sign are visible in the basal segments (MIP).

Differential Diagnosis

Cystic fibrosis	– Generalized bronchiectasis (more often in the upper lobes than lower lobes) – Mucoid impaction – Hereditary disorder
Common variable immunodeficiency (CVID)	– Immunodeficiency with recurrent pneumonia, bronchiectasis, and chronic sinusitis
Yellow nail syndrome	– Recurrent bronchopulmonary infections – Bronchiectasis – Hypogammaglobulinemia – Yellow nails

Selected References

Nadel HR et al. The immotile cilia syndrome: radiological manifestations. Radiology 1985; 154: 651–655

Definition

▶ **Epidemiology**
Infants and young children are most often affected.

▶ **Etiology, pathophysiology, pathogenesis**
In adults the disorder is a sequela of difficulty swallowing from a variety of causes (neurologic, tumor-related, etc.) • The bronchial obstruction leads to atelectasis or, in the presence of a valve mechanism, to local hyperinflation.

Imaging Signs

▶ **Modality of choice**
Chest radiographs (on inspiration and expiration) • Lateral view of pharynx and neck • CT may be needed to verify and localize radiographic findings.

▶ **Radiographic and CT findings**
Complete bronchial obstruction without collateral air drift leads to atelectasis • Stenosis with a valve mechanism leads to hyperinflation • Obstruction without a valve mechanism may appear normal or may lead to recurrent infiltrates • Foreign bodies with a distinct shadow are found in only 10% of cases • CT directly visualizes intraluminal foreign bodies.

▶ **Pathognomonic findings**
Unilateral hyperinflation with signs of a mass (mediastinal shift, unilateral low-lying diaphragmatic crus).

Clinical Aspects

▶ **Typical presentation**
Retching • Cough • Stridor • Cyanosis • Hypoxemia • Occasionally loss of consciousness.

▶ **Therapeutic options**
Bronchoscopic extraction of the foreign body.

▶ **Course and prognosis**
Prognosis is good with prompt removal of the foreign body • Delayed diagnosis can result in recurrent infections.

▶ **What does the clinician want to know?**
Diagnosis • Location.

Differential Diagnosis

Hyperinflation and/or hypertransradiant hemithorax	– No signs of a mass – No history
Atelectasis from other causes	– No aspiration event – Tumor obstruction

Fig. 2.16 Aspiration of a peanut. Increased transradiancy of the left lung with right mediastinal shift and flattened, caudally shifted left diaphragmatic crus.

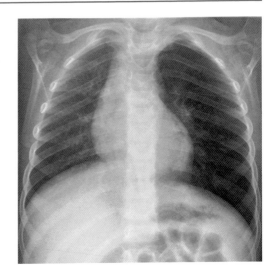

Tips and Pitfalls

Where the history is known, the diagnosis is straightforward • *Note:* In patients in whom aspiration is strongly suspected, bronchoscopy is indicated—even in the presence of negative radiographic findings.

Selected References

Wunsch R, Wunsch C, Darge K. [Fremdkörperaspiration.] Radiologe 1999; 39: 467–471 [In German]

Definition

▶ **Epidemiology**
Mainly existing cases; occupational safety regulations have greatly reduced the incidence of new cases • Chronic inhalation of inorganic dusts (especially silicate in crystalline form) • Long-term exposure (sand blasters, quarry workers, miners).

▶ **Etiology, pathophysiology, pathogenesis**
Alveolar phagocytosis and interstitial deposition of inhaled particles • Development of interstitial reticulonodular granulomas of varying severity up to and including massive fibrosis. • This leads to parenchymal shrinkage and scarring with emphysema.

Imaging Signs

▶ **Modality of choice**
Radiographs, CT.

▶ **Radiographic findings**
Sharply demarcated, focal nodular lesions (1–10 mm in diameter) in the upper and middle lung fields, often with calcifications • These may become confluent, forming massive conglomerates • Hilar and mediastinal lymph nodes show eggshell calcification.

▶ **CT findings**
Micronodular lesions in the center and at the periphery of a lobule within the upper and middle lung fields • Signs of pulmonary fibrosis.

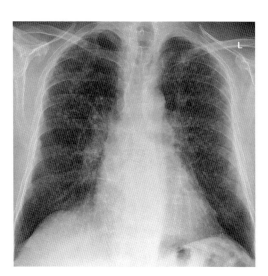

Fig. 3.1 Anthracosilicosis in a 64-year-old man. Sharply demarcated, relatively dense, and partially confluent focal nodular lesions disseminated over both lungs, and increasing from base to apex. Bilateral apicolateral pleural calluses. Perihilar shadowing.

Fig. 3.2 Anthracosilicosis in a 60-year-old man. The plain chest radiograph (**a**) and axial CT scans (**c, d**) show sharply demarcated nodules and large scarred focal lesions (conglomerates) in the upper lung fields, accompanied by shortening of the hila. CT also demonstrates bullous formations. The enlarged, severely calcified hilar and mediastinal lymph nodes, some exhibiting eggshell calcification, are best visualized on the coronal MIP (**b**).

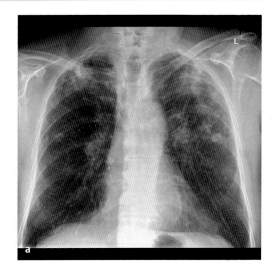

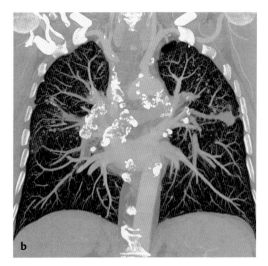

Fig. 3.2 c, d

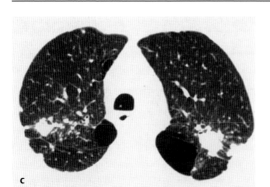

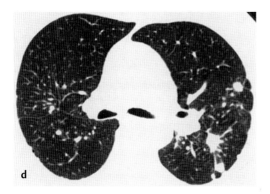

▶ **Pathognomonic findings**
Symmetric micronodular changes in the upper and middle lung fields • Calluses.

Clinical Aspects

▶ **Typical presentation**
Dyspnea at rest and during exercise • Cough • Cyanosis • Progressive fibrosis can lead to right heart failure.

▶ **Therapeutic options**
Discontinue exposure • Antiobstructive medication.

▶ **Course and prognosis**
Disease may progress even without continued exposure • Life expectancy in uncomplicated pneumoconiosis is normal but is reduced in the presence of progressive fibrosis.

▶ **What does the clinician want to know?**
Diagnosis and differential diagnosis. • Distinguish uncomplicated from complicated forms.

Differential Diagnosis

Sarcoidosis	– Can have identical radiographic morphology
	– No history of occupational exposure
	– Typical laboratory findings
Langerhans cell histiocytosis	– Cystic changes
	– No lymphadenopathy

Tips and Pitfalls

Radiographically indistinguishable from sarcoidosis; history of occupational exposure is crucial for the diagnosis.

Selected References

Bergin CJ et al. CT in silicosis: Correlation with plain films and pulmonary function tests. AJR Am J Roentgenol 1986; 146: 477–483

Hoffmeyer F et al. [Pneumokoniosen.] Pneumologie 2007; 61: 774–797 [In German]

Remy-Jardin M et al. Coal workers pneumoconiosis: CT assessment in exposed workers and correlation with radiographic findings. Radiology 1990; 177: 363–371

Definition

Pneumoconiosis caused by fibrous mineral silicates.

▶ **Epidemiology**
Occupational disease • Manifests after 20–40 years of chronic exposure.

▶ **Etiology, pathophysiology, pathogenesis**
Inhalation of asbestos fibers (20–150 μm) • Deposition of fibers in the pulmonary parenchyma leads to foreign body reaction with proliferation of nodular connective tissue • Disseminated alveolar septal and peribronchiolar fibrosis • Dose–response relationship • Asbestos-associated changes include pleural plaques.

Imaging Signs

▶ **Modality of choice**
CT.

▶ **Radiographic and CT findings**
Findings are variable and may be normal • Streaky and reticular shadowing primarily in the basal segments • Linear opacities and parenchymal bands parallel to the pleura • Platelike and round areas of atelectasis • Honeycombing • Scarring with emphysema • Bronchiectasis • Pleural plaques • Recurrent pleural effusions.

▶ **Pathognomonic findings**
None • Bridging symptoms such as calcified pleural plaques and a history of occupational exposure are crucial to the diagnosis.

Clinical Aspects

▶ **Typical presentation**
Initially there is often an asymptomatic effusion • Symptoms often occur only 20 years after exposure and include a restrictive ventilation defect with an obstructive component • Asbestos bodies in the sputum.

▶ **Therapeutic options**
Symptomatic supportive treatment.

▶ **Course and prognosis**
Progressive pneumoconiosis even after exposure has been discontinued • Complications include pulmonary fibrosis • Risk of lung cancer is 50 times higher in smokers with chronic exposure • Pleural mesothelioma.

▶ **What does the clinician want to know?**
Extent of findings • International Labour Office classification • Tumor development.

Fig. 3.3 Asbestos-associated changes in a 70-year-old man. Circumscribed, irregular streaky reticular changes in the right basal subpleural region. (**a**) Bridging symptom with right anterior and posterior paravertebral pleural calcifications (arrow).

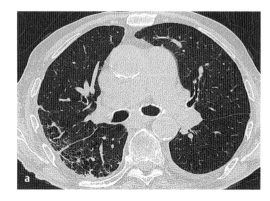

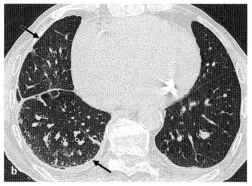

Differential Diagnosis

Idiopathic pulmonary fibrosis	– Comparable interstitial fibrosis
	– Ground-glass opacities are more common
	– No pleural plaques
Scleroderma	– Finely reticular interstitial shadowing
	– No pleural plaques
	– Esophageal dilation
Rheumatism	– No pleural plaques
	– Joint pathology
	– Known underlying disease
Postinfectious or posttraumatic pleural thickening	– Calluses are shaped differently and occur at other locations
	– History

Tips and Pitfalls

A causal relationship is difficult to establish in the absence of chronic asbestos exposure.

Selected References

Chong S et al. Pneumoconiosis: Comparison of imaging and pathologic findings. Radiographics 2006; 26: 59–77
Kim K et al. Imaging of occupational lung disease. Radiographics 2001; 21: 1371–1391
Merget R. [Pneumokoniosen.] Pneumologe 2006; 3: 450–460 [In German]

Definition

Pneumonia acquired in normal, daily life.

▶ **Epidemiology**

Diagnostic microbiologic evaluation is carried out in less than 30% of cases of community-acquired pneumonia; the pathogen can be positively identified in only 5% of cases • Pneumococci (*Streptococcus pneumoniae*), *Mycoplasma pneumoniae, Haemophilus influenzae, Chlamydia pneumoniae*, and viruses (adenovirus, respiratory syncytial virus) are the most common pathogens; less common pathogens include *Legionella pneumophila, Staphylococcus aureus, Klebsiella pneumoniae* • Protozoans and fungi are practically never the cause • The spectrum of pathogens varies depending on seasonal, geographic, socioeconomic, and intrinsic factors (age, comorbidity).

▶ **Etiology, pathophysiology, pathogenesis**

These depend on the pathogen. Pneumococci, *Klebsiella, Legionella*, and *Mycoplasma* typically cause lobar consolidation. *Haemophilus influenzae* and staphylococci cause bronchopneumonic infiltrates, and viruses and mycoplasmas cause interstitial or mixed interstitial-alveolar infiltrates.

Imaging Signs

▶ **Modality of choice**

Radiographs • CT is indicated only where findings are equivocal or there is clinical suspicion but no radiographic correlate.

▶ **Radiographic findings**

Homogeneous, nonsegmental area of opacification with a pleural interface and alveolar and/or lobar infiltrates • Ill-defined focal heterogeneous opacities in a segmental configuration with bronchopneumonic infiltrates.

▶ **CT findings**

Findings are similar to radiography • CT is more sensitive in detecting associated findings (multifocal manifestation, pleuritis, liquefaction).

▶ **Pathognomonic findings**

See "Radiographic findings."

Clinical Aspects

▶ **Typical presentation**

Fever, cough, dyspnea, sputum, chest pain, poor general health • Leukocytosis with leftward shift • It is usually not possible to identify the pathogen as noninvasive diagnostic evaluation (sputum analysis) is inefficient and delayed.

▶ **Therapeutic options**

Antibiotics (empirical therapy).

▶ **Course and prognosis**

Manifestation and course depend on the specific patient and the infecting pathogen (comorbidities and virulence, respectively) • Uncomplicated disease resolves completely.

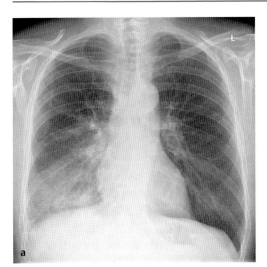

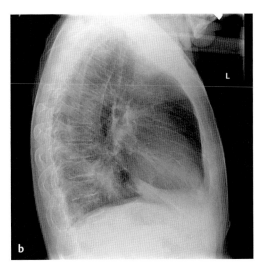

Fig. 4.1 Community-acquired pneumonia in a 55-year-old man. Typical findings in lobar pneumonia. Homogeneous area of infiltrate in the right lower lobe with broad pleural contact. Slight pleural effusion.

▶ **What does the clinician want to know?**
Confirmation of tentative diagnosis of pneumonia ● Extent of findings.

Differential Diagnosis

Radiographic findings alone cannot point to a specific causative pathogen. However, this is not necessary as clinical and radiographic findings are together only suggestive and empirical treatment regimens are available.

Tips and Pitfalls

When imaging findings are interpreted in conjunction with clinical data, findings are usually suggestive ● Radiographic findings are negative in this regard in about one-third of patients with clinically suspected pneumonia ● Usually these cases are severe, clinically relevant respiratory infections.

Selected References

Franquet T. Imaging of pneumonia: trends and algorithm. Eur Resp J 2001; 18: 196–208
Herold CJ, Sailer JG. Community-acquired and nosocomial pneumonias. Eur Radiol 2004; 14 (Suppl. 3): E2–E20
Traver RD et al. Radiology of community acquired pneumonia. Radiol Clin North Am 2005; 43: 497–512
Washington L, Palacio D. Imaging of bacterial pulmonary infection in the immunocompetent patient. Semin Roentgenol 2007; 42: 122–145

Definition

Pneumonia acquired in a treatment facility.

▶ **Epidemiology**

Estimated prevalence in intensive care units is 10–50% • Pathogens predominantly include both Gram-negative pathogens (*Pseudomonas aeruginosa, Klebsiella* ssp., Enterobacteriaceae, *Proteus* ssp., *Escherichia coli, Serratia marcescens*) and Gram-positive cocci (*Streptococcus pneumoniae, Staphylococcus aureus*), *Legionella*, and viruses • Mixed infections are common • Despite intensive serologic, immunologic, and microbiologic diagnostic testing, a specific pathogen can be identified in only about one-third of all cases (it can be difficult to distinguish infection from contamination).

▶ **Etiology, pathophysiology, pathogenesis**

There are several reasons for the high prevalence • Patient-related factors include age, immune status, a previous or underlying disorder, and aspiration • Risks related to treatments include breaching of physiologic barriers by intubation and artificial respiration, catheters, and antacid medications • Environmental risks include staff and other patients.

Imaging Signs

▶ **Modality of choice**

Radiographs • CT is indicated only where findings are equivocal or to rule out other pathology.

▶ **Radiographic and CT findings**

There is a broad spectrum of infiltrative changes, which depend on the risk factors. Changes may be focal, unilocular, multilocular, or may include pleural effusion • Note that repeated follow-up examinations are indicated not only to confirm or exclude complications but also for diagnostic purposes as it is difficult to predict when infiltrates may occur • Findings on radiographs obtained too early (within a few hours of the onset of clinical symptoms) or in a neutropenic patient may initially be negative.

▶ **Pathognomonic findings**

See the various forms of pneumonia for specific findings.

Clinical Aspects

▶ **Typical presentation**

Hospitalized patients with multiple disorders may not always show typical symptoms pointing to pneumonia. Therefore diagnostic radiography has a particularly important role in excluding other foci of infection.

▶ **Therapeutic options**

Specific antibiotics in patients in whom the pathogen has been isolated or empirical treatment for those in whom this is not possible.

Infections

Fig. 4.2 Hospital-acquired pneumonia in a 57-year-old woman (*Pneumocystis* pneumonia and fungal pneumonia secondary to perforation of the sigmoid colon). The plain chest radiographs show extensive nodular confluent infiltrates in both lungs with much of the opacity consisting of acinar nodules. The peripheral subpleural parenchymal segments have largely been spared. There was no pleural effusion or lymphadenopathy.

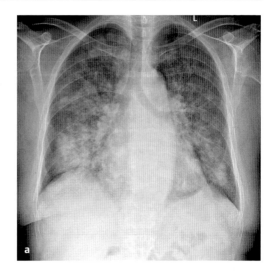

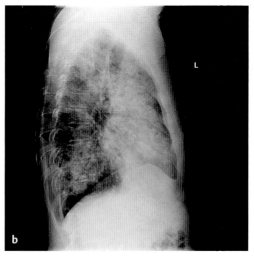

▶ **Course and prognosis**

Mortality has been cited at 20–50%.

▶ **What does the clinician want to know?**

Confirm or exclude pneumonia ● Extent of findings ● Follow-up ● Complications.

Differential Diagnosis

Comorbidities may render clinical and radiologic diagnosis and differential diagnosis difficult ● Even where history and clinical data are considered, the accuracy of diagnostic radiography in intensive care patients is only about 50%.

Atelectasis	– Volume loss
	– No constellation of infection
	– May be in a specific location in bedridden patients (supine)
Aspiration pneumonia	– History
	– Located in the posterobasal segments
	– Predilection for the right side
Pulmonary embolism or infarct	– Clinical aspects
	– No constellation of infection
Atypical edema	– Patients with heart failure and pre-existing pulmonary disease (emphysema or chronic obstructive pulmonary disease) or pulmonary embolism can develop localized atypical edema that mimics pneumonia
	– Clinical findings and rapid resolution with re-established cardiac compensation are diagnostic
ARDS	– History and clinical findings

Tips and Pitfalls

Reliable diagnostic findings that rule out other pathology can only be obtained by evaluating imaging data in conjunction with clinical data.

Selected References

Franquet T. Imaging of pneumonia: trends and algorithm. Eur Resp J 2001; 18: 196–208

Herold CJ, Sailer JG. Community-acquired and nosocomial pneumonias. Eur Radiol 2004; 14 (Suppl. 3): E2 – E20

Washington L, Palacio D. Imaging of bacterial pulmonary infection in the immunocompetent patient. Semin Roentgenol 2007; 42: 122–145

Definition

Pneumonia related to pathogens in immunocompromised patients (pneumonia caused by microorganisms that occur only in patients with immune deficiency or receiving immunosuppressants but not in immunocompetent persons).

▶ **Epidemiology**

The spectrum of pathogens includes the bacteria, viruses, fungi, and protozoans that colonize the oropharynx and airways in immunocompetent persons as saprophytes without causing infection • The type and severity of the immune defect influence the spectrum of pathogens that may be expected • The spectrum of pathogens after organ transplantation varies over time • In HIV-infected patients the risk of pulmonary infection depends on the number of CD4 cells: > 200/μL, bacteria; < 200/μL, *Pneumocystis jirovecii*, fungi, adenoviruses, RNA viruses, herpesviruses, influenza viruses; < 100/μL, cytomegalovirus, atypical mycobacteria.

▶ **Etiology, pathophysiology, pathogenesis**

The constellation of pathogens in neutropenia (steroid therapy, induction therapy in acute myeloid leukemia, bone marrow transplantation) includes bacteria, fungi (*Aspergillus, Mucoraceae, Candida*) • Pathogens in B-cell dysfunction (lymphoproliferative disorders, bone marrow transplantation, chemotherapy) include bacteria (pneumococci, *Haemophilus influenzae, Klebsiella, Pseudomonas, Neisseria*) • Pathogens in T-cell dysfunction (lymphoproliferative disorders; chemotherapy; bone marrow, stem cell, lung, heart, liver, or kidney transplantation; steroid therapy; HIV infection; infection with immunomodulatory viruses such as cytomegalovirus, Epstein-Barr virus, varicella zoster virus) include bacteria, mycobacteria, *Listeria*, cryptococci, *P. jirovecii* and other fungi, protozoans, and viruses.

Imaging Signs

▶ **Modality of choice**

Radiographs and CT • CT is superior to conventional radiographs in terms of sensitivity and specificity and is often indicated for this reason.

▶ **Radiographic and CT findings**

These depend on the underlying disorder, risk factors, immunocompetence, and type of pathogen (see that section).

▶ **Pathognomonic findings**

See the various forms of pneumonia.

Clinical Aspects

▶ **Typical presentation**

The typical constellation of findings associated with pneumonia (rise in temperature, increased blood count, abnormal C-reactive protein, physical findings) may not be present in the early stages or findings may be uncharacteristic • Symptoms depend on the individual patient's immunocompetence and the virulence of the pathogen • Radiographic findings represent a crucial diagnostic adjunct to immunologic and serologic studies.

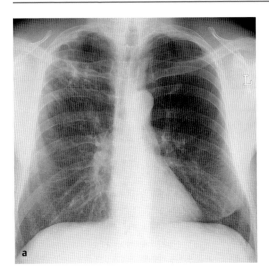

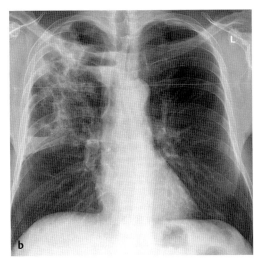

Fig. 4.3 Opportunistic pneumonia in a 53-year-old man with HIV infection (CD4 > 500/μL). The images were obtained only 2 weeks apart. The initial, not very extensive, infiltrate around the right upper lobe (**a**) rapidly developed into necrotizing pneumonia with abscess formation (**b**) as clinical findings worsened. Extensive diagnostic testing failed to identify the pathogen (*Chlamydia*, mycoplasmas, *P. jirovecii*, and mycobacteria were excluded).

▶ **Therapeutic options**
Prompt treatment has a decisive influence on the prognosis.

▶ **Course and prognosis**
Mortality is as high as 50 % in severe cases involving respiratory or circulatory insufficiency, extent, or rapid progression.

▶ **What does the clinician want to know?**
Confirmation of a tentative diagnosis of pneumonia ● Extent of findings ● Follow-up ● Complications ● Narrow down the spectrum of possible pathogens.

Differential Diagnosis

Experience and knowledge of the type and severity of the immune defect are crucial in narrowing down the spectrum of possible pathogens ● Specific constellations of radiographic findings provide useful diagnostic information in this context (this applies especially to pulmonary mycosis and mycobacterial infection) ● However, mixed forms are common.

Extrapulmonary infections	– Infections of the gastrointestinal tract, urinary tract, paranasal sinuses, and central nervous system must be excluded
Edema, hemorrhage, infarct, ARDS, etc.	– Reliable differential diagnosis is not possible without clinical information

Tips and Pitfalls

When interpreted in conjunction with clinical data, findings are usually suggestive ● Where such data are unavailable, it will not be possible to reliably distinguish pneumonia from other pathology.

Selected References

Franquet T. Imaging of pneumonia: trends and algorithm. Eur Resp J 2001; 18: 196–208
Gharib AM, Stern EJ. Radiology of pneumonia. Med Clin North Am 2001; 85: 1461–1491
Tuengerthal S. [Radiologie der opportunistischen Pneumonien.] Radiologe 2005; 45: 373–384 [In German]

Definition

▶ **Epidemiology**
A fundamental distinction should be drawn between community-acquired and hospital-acquired (nosocomial) pneumonias as different spectra of pathogens must be considered • Typical pathogens in lobar pneumonia include pneumococci, *Klebsiella*, and *Proteus* • Mycoplasmas and *Legionella* can produce a similar picture.

▶ **Etiology, pathophysiology, pathogenesis**
The disorder develops in the distal air spaces where gas exchange occurs • It progresses in pathoanatomic stages: Red hepatization with an erthyrocytic exudate • Gray hepatization with influx of leukocytes • Yellow hepatization with proteolytic breakdown of the exudate.

Imaging Signs

▶ **Modality of choice**
Radiographs • CT is indicated only where findings are equivocal or there is clinical suspicion but no radiographic correlate.

▶ **Radiographic findings**
Homogeneous, nonsegmental area of opacification with a pleural interface consistent with initial manifestation in the distal air spaces • Air bronchogram • Lobar borders are intact • Usually there is no volume change, although expansion may occur ("bulging fissure" sign) • Findings and course depend on the individual patient's immunocompetence and the virulence of the pathogen.

▶ **CT findings**
Findings are similar to radiography • CT is more sensitive in detecting associated findings (multifocal manifestation, pleuritis, liquefaction).

▶ **Pathognomonic findings**
See "Radiographic findings."

Clinical Aspects

▶ **Typical presentation**
Antibiotics have made the typical clinical picture (acute onset with chills, fever, tachycardia, tachypnea, cough with rusty brown sputum, chest pain, and very poor general health) less common • Blood count shows leukocytosis with left shift • Manifestation and course of the pneumonia depend on the individual patient's immunocompetence and the virulence of the pathogen.

▶ **Therapeutic options**
Antibiotics • In hospital-acquired infections in particular an antibiotic sensitivity study to isolate the pathogen is indicated.

▶ **Course and prognosis**
Uncomplicated disease resolves completely although this can take weeks to months • Possible complications include pulmonary abscess, empyema, and septic embolism.

Fig. 4.4   Lobar pneumonia. The plain chest radiographs show two homogeneous areas of infiltrate with broad pleural contact in the posterior right upper lobe and right middle lobe. Associated with it is a slight pneumothorax with fluid accumulation.

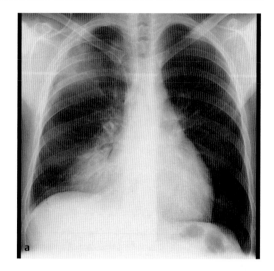

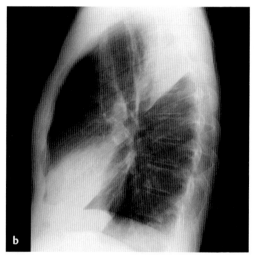

▶ **What does the clinician want to know?**
Confirmation of a tentative diagnosis of pneumonia ● Degree of severity ● Complicating findings ● Follow-up ● Only rarely will the radiologist be asked to narrow the spectrum of possible pathogens as the treatment of acute community-acquired pneumonia is empirical and does not require identification of a specific pathogen.

Differential Diagnosis

Morphologic findings on the radiograph alone do not provide evidence of a specific pathogen; at best they can be used to differentiate between bacterial and viral pneumonia ● Correlation of imaging findings with history and clinical data is essential for the diagnosis ● Experience is a useful guide: viral infections are most common in children, mycoplasma pneumonia in adolescents, and bacterial pneumonia in adults.

Pulmonary embolism or infarct	– Clinical aspects – No constellation of infection
Bronchial carcinoma with poststenotic pneumonia	– CT and bronchoscopy are indicated where clinical or radiographic findings suggest such a lesion (findings refractive to treatment or recurring at the same location)
Atypical edema	– Patients with left heart failure can develop localized atypical edema that mimics pneumonia – Clinical findings and rapid resolution with re-established cardiac compensation are diagnostic

Tips and Pitfalls

When interpreted in conjunction with clinical data, findings are usually suggestive ● The differentiation between lobar pneumonia, bronchopneumonia, and interstitial pneumonia is not always helpful as the same pathogen can produce widely varying pictures.

Selected References

Franquet T. Imaging of pneumonia: trends and algorithm. Eur Resp J 2001; 18: 196–208
Herold CJ, Sailer JG. Community-acquired and nosocomial pneumonias. Eur Radiol 2004; 14 (Suppl. 3): E2–E20
Washington L, Palacio D. Imaging of bacterial pulmonary infection in the immunocompetent patient. Semin Roentgenol 2007; 42: 122–145

Definition

▶ **Epidemiology**
A fundamental distinction should be made between community-acquired and hospital-acquired (nosocomial) pneumonias as different pathogens must be considered • Typical pathogens include staphylococci, streptococci, *Pseudomonas*, and anaerobes • *Haemophilus*, mycoplasmas, and viruses can produce a similar picture.

▶ **Etiology, pathophysiology, pathogenesis**
The infection begins in the bronchioles (often secondary to viral infection of the upper respiratory tract) and spreads to the peribronchial alveoli • The disease does not progress in stages, rather findings include the simultaneous presence of acute and resolving infiltrates.

Imaging Signs

▶ **Modality of choice**
Radiographs • CT is indicated only where findings are equivocal or there is clinical suspicion but no radiographic correlate.

▶ **Radiographic findings**
Ill-defined, heterogeneous infiltrates often showing a focal pattern • Segmental configuration • An air bronchogram is usually absent • Mucus obstruction of the airways produces subsegmental atelectasis, leading to volume loss • Abscesses • Findings and course depend on the individual patient's immunocompetence and the virulence of the pathogen.

▶ **CT findings**
Findings are similar to radiography • CT is more sensitive in detecting associated findings (multifocal manifestation, pleuritis, liquefaction).

▶ **Pathognomonic findings**
See "Radiographic findings."

Clinical Aspects

▶ **Typical presentation**
Subacute onset • Slowly increasing fever • Productive cough with mucopurulent sputum • Status of general health varies and may be only slightly impaired • Manifestation and course of the pneumonia depend on the individual patient's immunocompetence and the virulence of the pathogen.

▶ **Therapeutic options**
Antibiotics • In hospital-acquired infections in particular an antibiotic sensitivity study to isolate the pathogen is indicated.

▶ **Course and prognosis**
Uncomplicated cases have a good prognosis • Parenchymal necrosis results in residual scarring.

▶ **What does the clinician want to know?**
Confirmation of a tentative diagnosis of pneumonia • Narrow down the spectrum of possible pathogens.

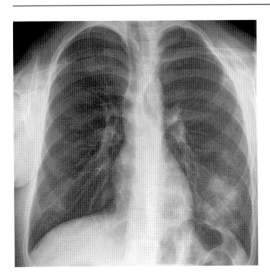

Fig. 4.5 Bronchopneumonia in a 17-year-old boy. The plain chest radiograph shows focal confluent infiltrates in the lower left lung field.

Differential Diagnosis

Morphologic findings on the radiograph alone do not provide evidence of a specific pathogen; at best they can be used to differentiate between bacterial and viral pneumonia ● Correlation of imaging findings with history and clinical data is essential to the diagnosis ● Experience is a useful guide: viral infections are most common in children, mycoplasma pneumonia in adolescents, and bacterial pneumonia in adults.

Lobar pneumonia, interstitial pneumonia	– Confluent lesions in bronchopneumonia can mimic lobar pneumonia – The differentiation between lobar pneumonia, bronchopneumonia, and interstitial pneumonia is not always helpful as the same pathogen can produce widely varying pictures

Tips and Pitfalls

When interpreted in conjunction with clinical data, findings are usually suggestive.

Selected References

Franquet T. Imaging of pneumonia: trends and algorithm. Eur Resp J 2001; 18: 196–208
Herold CJ, Sailer JG. Community-acquired and nosocomial pneumonias. Eur Radiol 2004; 14(Suppl. 3):E2–E20
Washington L, Palacio D. Imaging of bacterial pulmonary infection in the immunocompetent patient. Semin Roentgenol 2007; 42: 122–145

Definition

The term "atypical pneumonia" was, in the past, used to describe pneumonias with atypical clinical, laboratory, and radiologic findings • Today the term is applied to pneumonias in which the pathogen is difficult to isolate.

▶ **Epidemiology**

Affected patients include those with chronic wasting diseases, those on long-term antibiotic therapy, or those with primary or secondary immunodeficiency (cytostatic agents, immunosuppressives) • Typical pathogens include *Pneumocystis jirovecii*, viruses, fungi, chlamydiae, and rickettsiae.

▶ **Etiology, pathophysiology, pathogenesis**

Nonbacterial pneumonia • Infection develops in and is largely limited to the interstitium with minimal involvement of the alveolar parenchyma, i.e., with minimal mixed interstitial-alveolar infiltrates • Capillary damage leads to hemorrhagic interstitial and/or alveolar edema.

Imaging Signs

▶ **Modality of choice**

Radiographs • CT is indicated only where findings are equivocal or there is clinical suspicion but no radiographic correlate.

▶ **Radiographic and CT findings**

Bilateral symmetric linear, reticular, or reticulonodular opacities and/or ground-glass opacities • Often there is mixed interstitial-alveolar shadowing • Findings and course depend on the individual patient's immunocompetence and the virulence of the pathogen.

▶ **Pathognomonic findings**

See radiographic and CT findings.

Clinical Aspects

▶ **Typical presentation**

Insidious onset with moderate fever without chills, nonproductive cough, flulike headache and joint pain • Blood count shows slight leukocytosis with relative lymphocytosis • Clinical findings and course depend on the individual patient's immunocompetence and the virulence of the pathogen.

▶ **Therapeutic options**

The pathogen must be isolated to permit specific therapy • Where indicated, immunocompetence should be improved by treating the underlying disorder.

▶ **Course and prognosis**

With effective therapy the disease resolves completely.

▶ **What does the clinician want to know?**

Confirmation of a tentative diagnosis of pneumonia and characterization.

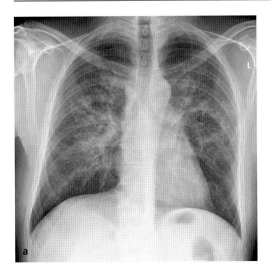

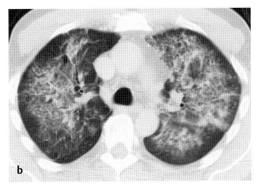

Fig. 4.6 Interstitial pneumonia in a 50-year-old man with Wegener granulomatosis, clinical picture of fever with headache, extremity pain, and productive cough with brown sputum following travel in the tropics.

a The plain chest radiograph shows interstitial shadowing limited primarily to the mid-lung with secondary opacity and masking of vascular structures.

b CT findings include ground-glass opacity and reticular shadowing. The peripheral subpleural parenchymal segments have largely been spared (extensive diagnostic testing failed to identify the pathogen).

Differential Diagnosis

Morphologic findings on the radiograph alone do not provide evidence of a specific pathogen; at best they can be used to differentiate between bacterial and viral pneumonia • Correlation of imaging findings with history and clinical data is essential for the diagnosis • Experience is a useful guide: viral infections are most common in children, mycoplasma pneumonia in adolescents, and bacterial pneumonia in adults.

Mycoplasma pneumonia	– Most common community-acquired pneumonia – Symptoms are relatively mild compared with radiographic findings; initially there are interstitial infiltrates, later followed by segmental alveolar infiltrates; pleural effusion and lymphadenopathy are rare
Pneumocystis pneumonia	– Most common atypical pneumonia in immunocompromised patients – Radiographic findings are negative in 10% of cases, CT invariably positive: bilateral perihilar and basal interstitial shadowing progressing to edemalike alveolar infiltrates – Pentamidine prophylaxis results in atypical findings: upper lobe redistribution, cystic changes
Cytomegalovirus pneumonia	– Opportunistic infection, usually endogenous reactivation – Radiograph shows bilateral ground-glass opacity (resembling edema) merging with multifocal consolidations
Fungal pneumonia	– Opportunistic infection – Unspecific clinical findings – Radiographs and CT show solitary or multiple focal infiltrates with a halo with or without liquefaction
Chlamydia pneumonia	– Community-acquired – Clinical findings include pharyngitis, fever, unproductive cough; self-limiting – Unspecific radiographic findings; indistinguishable from bacterial pneumonias
Rickettsia pneumonia	– Fever, cough, myalgia, joint pain – Unspecific radiographic findings; infiltrates resemble pneumonia or bronchopneumonia and often resolve slowly
Nontuberculous mycobacterial Infection	– 20% of all cases do not exhibit the classic form with nodular changes and irregular interstitial bands primarily in the middle lobe or lingula segments

Tips and Pitfalls

Broad differential diagnosis • Imaging findings are not usually helpful in identifying the spectrum of pathogens • The differentiation between lobar pneumonia, bronchopneumonia, and interstitial pneumonia is not always helpful as the same pathogen can produce widely varying pictures.

Selected References

Franquet T. Imaging of pneumonia: trends and algorithm. Eur Resp J 2001; 18: 196–208
Tuengerthal S. [Radiologie der opportunistischen Pneumonien.] Radiologe 2005; 45: 373–384 [In German]

Definition

▶ **Epidemiology**
Damage instigated by liquid or solid substances as opposed to airborne substances ● Risk factors include infancy (foreign body aspiration), disorientation, sedation, difficulty swallowing (neurogenic or postoperative), reflux, vomiting, alcoholism.

▶ **Etiology, pathophysiology, pathogenesis**
Aspiration pneumonia is pneumonia resulting from aspiration of infectious material (mucus from the upper respiratory and digestive tract, often but not invariably anaerobes) ● Aspiration pneumonitis is an inflammatory reaction to chemical toxins secondary to aspiration of gastric juice or other noxious agents.

Imaging Signs

▶ **Modality of choice**
Radiographs and CT.

▶ **Radiographic and CT findings**
Findings are variable and depend on the type and quantity of the aspirate, frequency of aspiration, patient position, and the body's reaction:
- Bland aspirated material causes nodular shadowing for 24 hours, which CT shows to be intraluminal ● A "tree-in-bud" sign may be present.
- Aspirated gastric juice causes shadowing and can progress to ARDS.
  Aspirated infectious material causes pneumonia and can lead to formation of an abscess.
- Chronic or recurrent aspiration can lead to bronchiectasis in the affected segments.
- Location varies with position ● Upright = basal segments of the lower lobes with predilection for the right side ● Supine = posterior upper lobe and apical segment of the lower lobe.

Clinical Aspects

▶ **Typical presentation**
Symptoms in acute aspiration include cough, shortness of breath, tachypnea, and others ● Resembles acute coronary syndrome ● Symptoms in chronic recurrent aspiration resemble those of asthma.

▶ **Course and prognosis**
Depend on the pathogenetic mechanism and/or predisposing factors and risks.

▶ **What does the clinician want to know?**
Depends on the pathogenetic mechanism: Identify and localize the foreign body ● Complications.

Fig. 4.7 Aspiration in a 60-year-old man following irradiation of an oropharyngeal carcinoma.

a Initial findings after aspiration include streaky and patchy opacities in the right middle and lower lobes.

b Within 3 days, aspiration pneumonia developed—manifested as massive opacification of the right lower lobe.

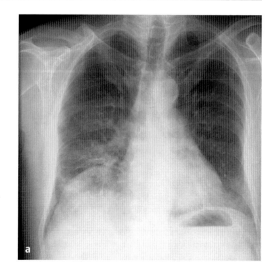

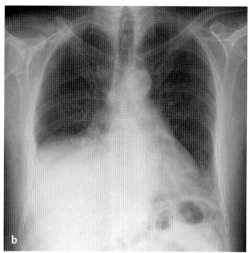

Differential Diagnosis

Consolidations in segments at risk of aspiration	– All types of inflammatory and noninflammatory disorders (pneumonia, chronic obstructive pulmonary disease, collagen and vascular disorders, bronchioalveolar carcinoma, pulmonary sequestration, etc.) – Diagnosis and differential diagnosis depends on clinical findings

Tips and Pitfalls

In patients in whom the history does not suggest aspiration, the cause of the pathology is often not accurately diagnosed ● Pulmonary changes secondary to aspiration are often sweepingly interpreted as aspiration pneumonia even in the absence of an infective etiology ● Aspiration lacking an obvious acute event may be misinterpreted as hospital-acquired pneumonia (10% of cases of hospital-acquired pneumonia are attributable to aspiration).

Selected References

Franquet T et al. Aspiration diseases: findings, pitfalls, and differential diagnosis. Radiographics 2000; 20: 673–685

Marik PE. Aspiration pneumonitis and aspiration pneumonia. N Engl J Med 2001; 344: 655–671

Mylotte JM, Goodnough S, Gould M. Pneumonia versus aspiration pneumonitis in nursing home residents: prospective application of a clinical algorithm. Am J Geriatr Soc 2005; 53: 755–761

Definition

▶ **Epidemiology**
Complications of severe infections such as sepsis, endocarditis, catheter sepsis, or in drug abuse • Most common pathogens include staphylococci, streptococci, fungi, and Gram-negative bacilli.

▶ **Etiology, pathophysiology, pathogenesis**
Sudden occlusion of the pulmonary artery flow tract by a bloodborne clot infected with bacteria • Infection then spreads to the adjacent lung tissue.

Imaging Signs

▶ **Modality of choice**
CT is preferable to plain radiography.

▶ **Radiographic and CT findings**
Multiple bilateral, moderately sharply demarcated nodules measuring up to 2 cm, located primarily in the peripheral and basal regions • Increasing cavitations develop as the disorder progresses • Disorder progresses in stages • A feeding vessel sign is observed in 65% of cases • There may be wedge-shaped subpleural infarcted areas.

▶ **Pathognomonic findings**
The rapidly changing radiologic findings include bilateral peripheral nodules that tend to develop cavitations quickly.

Clinical Aspects

▶ **Typical presentation**
Signs of underlying sepsis or endocarditis • Fever • Cough • Hemoptysis • Symptoms of hepatitis B.

▶ **Therapeutic options**
Antibiotics • Management of the source of infection.

▶ **Course and prognosis**
Depend on the underlying disorder • Complicating empyema occurs in up to 40% all cases.

Differential Diagnosis

Metastases	– Slower growth
	– No septic clinical syndrome
	– History of known malignancy
Fungal infection	– Ill-defined border
	– Varying degrees of severity
Thromboembolic disease	– Wedge-shaped pleural opacity
	– CTA

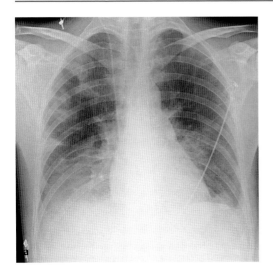

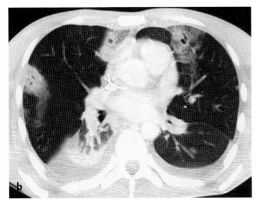

Fig. 4.8. Septic embolisms in a 25-year-old male drug addict.

a The plain chest radiograph was obtained at the bedside in a patient presenting with septic clinical syndrome. The film shows bilateral basal infiltrative changes, with a faint air bronchogram on the right. Other findings include small focal infiltrates, more pronounced on the right than on the left, some of which show focal transradiancies.

b CT confirms multiple septic embolisms along with an extensive pneumonic infiltrate in the right posterobasal region. There is slight bilateral pleural effusion.

Selected References

Huang RM et al. Septic pulmonary emboli: CT-radiographic correlation. AJR Am J Roentgenol 1989; 153: 41–45

Iwasaki Y et al. Spiral CT findings in septic pulmonary emboli. Eur J Radiol 2001; 37: 190–194

Definition

▶ **Epidemiology**
Common hospital-acquired pathogen • Found in infants and immunocompromised patients.
▶ **Etiology, pathophysiology, pathogenesis**
Airborne or hematogenous infection (look for focus) • Manifests itself as secondary bronchopneumonia or as primary staphylococcal pneumonia (especially in infants) • Tends to produce abscesses with cavitations • Pneumatoceles occur, especially in children • Pleural effusion and lymphadenopathy occur in 50% of all cases.

Imaging Signs

▶ **Modality of choice**
Radiographs, CT.
▶ **Radiographic and CT findings**
Focal infiltrates, such as occur in bronchopneumonia, often multilocular and bilateral • Hematogenous infections (from septic embolisms) are visualized as round or wedge-shaped foci • There may be vascular involvement (feeding vessel sign).
▶ **Pathognomonic findings**
Rapidly liquefying round focal infiltrates at multiple locations exhibiting rapid liquefaction and tending to form pneumatoceles (in children) and pleural empyemas.

Clinical Aspects

▶ **Typical presentation**
Fever with chills and chest pain • Blood-tinged purulent sputum.
▶ **Therapeutic options**
Antibiotics.
▶ **Course and prognosis**
Septic course following viral infection • Bronchiectasis occurs in chronic cases.
▶ **What does the clinician want to know?**
Complications: Abscesses, pyopneumothorax, empyema.

Differential Diagnosis

Round focal infiltrates with or without cavitations due to other causes	– Fungal pneumonia, Wegener granulomatosis, metastases, etc.
	– Can be readily differentiated due to the clinical picture of acute pneumonia.

Selected Reference

Webb WR, Higgins CB, eds. Thoracic imaging – Pulmonary and cardiovascular radiology. Philadelphia: William & Wilkins; 2005

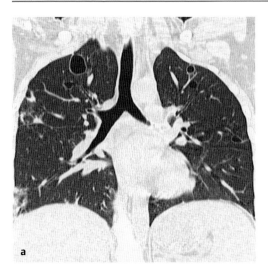

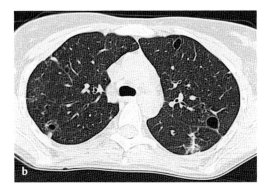

Fig. 4.9 Staphylococcal pneumonia in a 25-year-old woman with anorexia. Bilateral, multilocular liquefying infiltrates, some with a cystic appearance consistent with pneumatoceles.

Definition

▶ **Epidemiology**
Mycoplasma pneumoniae is a common pathogen that (along with pneumococci and viruses) causes community-acquired pneumonia in immunocompetent persons ● The disorder primarily affects children, adolescents, and young adults (patients 5–40 years old).

▶ **Etiology, pathophysiology, pathogenesis**
Infection is spread by droplet transmission with an incubation period of 10–20 days ● Primary interstitial pneumonia with peribronchiolar mononuclear cellular infiltrates and accompanying neutrophilic inflammatory reaction.

Imaging Signs

▶ **Modality of choice**
Radiographs.

▶ **Radiographic and CT findings**
Initially interstitial, later segmental or lobar acinar infiltrates (also appearing as ground-glass opacities on CT) ● Perihilar interstitial shadowing ● Rarely pleural effusion and/or lymphadenopathy (most common in children) ● Radiographic findings typically appear later than clinical findings.

▶ **Pathognomonic findings**
In contrast to the rather nonspecific clinical findings, imaging studies show extensive segmental or lobar infiltrates that resolve slowly.

Clinical Aspects

▶ **Typical presentation**
Fever ● Nonproductive cough ● Headache ● Flulike malaise ● Symptoms are relatively mild compared with the radiographic findings.

▶ **Therapeutic options**
Antibiotics (erythromycin, tetracyclines).

▶ **Course and prognosis**
Course is usually benign and self-limiting ● Bacterial superinfection or complications are rare.

▶ **What does the clinician want to know?**
Confirmation of tentative diagnosis of pneumonia.

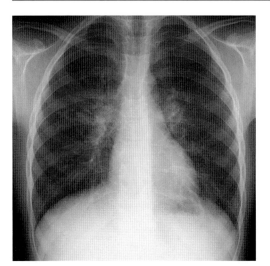

Fig. 4.10 Mycoplasma pneumonia in a 10-year-old boy. The plain chest radiograph shows significant bilateral, primarily perihilar interstitial shadowing with masking of vascular structures.

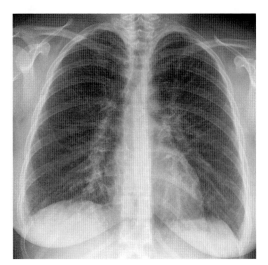

Fig. 4.11 Mycoplasma pneumonia in a 14-year-old girl with tachypnea, dyspnea, cough, and tachycardia. The plain chest radiograph shows bilateral, nearly symmetric, largely streaky interstitial shadowing extending into the periphery. No circumscribed infiltrates are detected. Associated bilateral effusion.

Differential Diagnosis

Chlamydial infection	– Usually indistinguishable as it produces similar clinical and radiographic symptoms
Bacterial pneumonias	– Different age group – Radiographic morphology varies with the pathogen
Opportunistic pneumonias	– Immunodeficiency – Risk groups
Aspiration pneumonia	– Clinical aspects – Risk factors (artificial respiration, fistula, etc.)

Tips and Pitfalls

It is easy to misjudge the response to therapy as radiographic findings typically resolve later than clinical symptoms.

Selected References

Finnegan OC, Fowler SJ, White RJ. Radiographic appearances of Mycoplasma pneumonia. Thorax 1981; 36: 469–472

Gückel C, Benz-Bohm G, Widemann B. Mycoplasmal pneumonias in childhood: roentgen features, differential diagnosis and review of literature. Pediatr Radiol 1989; 19: 499–503

Definition

▶ **Epidemiology**
Infection by *Mycobacterium tuberculosis* or, less often, *Mycobacterium bovis* ● The disease occurs worldwide but is more common in developing countries with a low socioeconomic standard; in developed countries it occurs primarily in immunocompromised patients (for example in individuals with AIDS).

▶ **Etiology, pathophysiology, pathogenesis**
Infection is spread by droplet transmission ● Infection initially spreads in the lung ● Hematogenous dissemination to other organs occurs but immunocompetent patients do not generally show extrathoracic manifestation.
  – *Primary tuberculosis* is the initial infection ● The cell-mediated immune response encapsulates the pathogen, forming caseous granulomas, usually in the middle or lower lobe ● The infection also involves the draining lymph nodes.
  – *Postprimary tuberculosis* is the reactivation of a latent infection (for example in immunosuppression) ● The infection usually arises from bacterial colonies in the vulnerable segments with high partial pressure of oxygen (apical and posterior segments of the upper lobe, apical segment of the lower lobe) ● In contrast to primary tuberculosis, the course is often progressive.

Imaging Signs

▶ **Modality of choice**
Radiographs, CT.

▶ **Radiographic and CT findings**
  – *Primary tuberculosis:* Findings are often normal ● Abnormal findings include variable alveolar shadowing that can cover the entire lobe and resolves slowly (within months) ● Pleural effusion (may be the only finding) ● Children often exhibit lymphadenopathy (CT shows central necrosis) with associated atelectasis ● Residual findings include a calcified pulmonary granuloma, or a granuloma with calcified hilar lymph nodes ● Cavitation or miliary seeding is rare and constitutes progressive primary tuberculosis.
  – *Postprimary tuberculosis:* Ill-defined infiltrates that show a predilection for the upper lobe ● Cavitation occurs in 20–45% of cases ● Endobronchial dissemination creates satellite foci and the "tree-in-bud" sign ● Hematogenous miliary dissemination of nodules measuring 1–2 mm may occur ● Bronchial involvement with thickening of the bronchial wall may occur ● The infection heals with scarring, leading to volume loss and bronchiectasis.
  – *Differentiating active from inactive tuberculosis:* This is difficult and requires previous imaging studies ● Constant findings over more than 6 months are inconsistent with activity ● Findings suggesting active tuberculosis include consolidations, bronchogenic spread ("tree-in-bud" sign), hematogenous miliary dissemination and cavitations ● Calcified foci and bronchiectasis suggest inactive tuberculosis.

Fig. 4.12 Active open pulmonary tuberculosis in a 31-year-old man with a 1-month history of fatigue, fever, and cough. The plain chest radiograph shows patchy, confluent infiltrates with small focal areas of liquefaction in the apical segment of the left lower lobe.

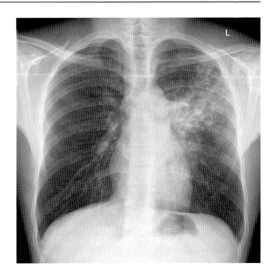

Fig. 4.13 Typical focal calcifications of healed tuberculosis in a 50-year-old woman. The plain chest radiograph shows focal calcifications of varying size in both lungs with no evidence of acute infiltrates. The left hilum is shortened and scarred.

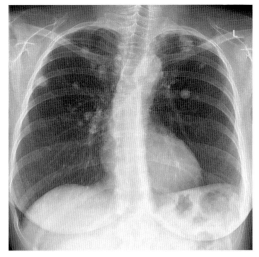

▶ **Pathognomonic findings**
  – *Primary tuberculosis:* Consolidation • Pleural effusion • Lymphadenopathy.
  – *Active versus inactive tuberculosis:* Cavitations showing a predilection for the upper lobe • Miliary tuberculosis.

Clinical Aspects

▶ **Typical presentation**
  – *Primary tuberculosis:* Children are often asymptomatic (cough and fever may be present) • Adults present with weight loss, limited exercise tolerance, fever, cough, hemoptysis.
  – *Postprimary tuberculosis:* Mild fever, night sweats, weight loss, limited exercise tolerance, and hemoptysis.
▶ **Therapeutic options**
  Antituberculous agents for at least 6 months (combined therapy with isoniazid, rifampicin, ethambutol, and pyrazinamide).
▶ **Course and prognosis**
  – *Primary tuberculosis* is usually self-limiting in immunocompetent patients • Progressive primary tuberculosis occurs in immunocompromised patients.
  – *Postprimary tuberculosis* is the reactivation of persisting pathogens and is usually associated with a progressive disorder • With adequate treatment and an intact immune system the disease will very often resolve completely • Patients with open tuberculosis should be kept in isolation.

Differential Diagnosis

Lobar pneumonia	– Tuberculosis persists longer and responds less well to treatment than lobar pneumonia
Chronic fungal infection	– Radiographic morphology is not clearly distinguishable from semi-invasive aspergillosis and other disorders
Sarcoidosis	– Can also exhibit primarily apical lung tissue changes and calcified lymph nodes

Tips and Pitfalls

The radiologic manifestation of tuberculosis is highly variable and can mimic other disorders; there is ample opportunity for misdiagnosis.

Selected References

Eisenhuber E et al. Radiologic diagnosis of lung tuberculosis. Radiologe 2007; 47: 393–400
Leung AN. Pulmonary tuberculosis: the essentials. Radiology 1999; 210: 307–322

Definition
....

▶ **Epidemiology**

Infection with nontuberculous mycobacteria, a group of about 20 different pathogens ● The most important bacteria that are facultatively pathogenic in humans include *Mycobacterium avium-intracellulare, kansasii*, and *abscessus.*

▶ **Etiology, pathophysiology, pathogenesis**

The pathogens are ubiquitous in soil and water ● Transmission occurs by inhalation or ingestion ● Chronically ill patients with risk factors (chronic obstructive pulmonary disease, bronchiectasis, cystic fibrosis, diabetes, alcoholism, AIDS) are affected most often.

Imaging Signs
....

▶ **Modality of choice**

Radiographs, CT.

▶ **Radiographic and CT findings**

– *M. avium-intracellulare* infection can assume one of three forms: The classic cavitary form resembles postprimary tuberculosis with infiltrates, cavitations, scarring, and nodular changes, showing a predilection for the upper lobe with endobronchial spread (older men, chronic obstructive pulmonary disease) ● The bronchiectatic nonclassic form includes bronchiectasis and centrilobular nodules primarily in the middle lobe and lingula segments (more common in elderly women, "Lady Windermere syndrome") ● Changes similar to those in hypersensitivity pneumonitis with nodular ground-glass opacities and ill-defined faint centrilobular nodules, air trapping ("hot tub lung").

– *M. kansasii* produces a pattern of involvement similar to postprimary tuberculosis.

– *M. abscessus* produces bronchiectasis and centrilobular nodules with a "tree-in-bud" sign ● Primarily affects the middle lobe and lingula segments.

▶ **Pathognomonic findings**

Findings are similar to postprimary tuberculosis ● However, pleural effusions are rare.

Clinical Aspects
....

▶ **Typical presentation**

Chronic cough ● Symptoms are often indistinguishable from those of tuberculosis.

▶ **Therapeutic options**

Combined therapy with macrolides, rifabutin, and ethambutol for over 6 months.

▶ **Course and prognosis**

This depends on the pattern of involvement and the patient's immunocompetence.

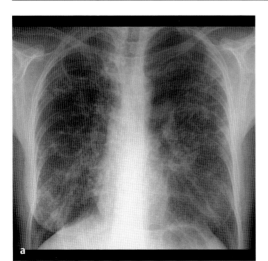

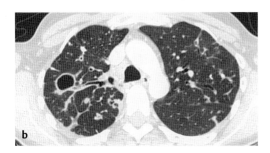

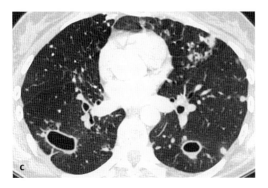

Fig. 4.14 Nontuberculous mycobacterial infection (*Mycobacterium malmoense*) in a 43-year-old woman. The plain chest radiograph and CT show bilateral thin-walled cavitations. Other findings include disseminated, partially clustered nodular lesions of varying size along with partial thickening of bronchial wall and bronchiectatic changes.

Differential Diagnosis

Tuberculosis	– Radiographic morphology not clearly distinguishable from nontuberculous mycobacterial infection
Pulmonary mycotic infection, especially chronic forms	– Usually multilocular focal infiltrates with or without cavitation or halo – Chronic pulmonary mycotic infections can also produce a picture resembling mycobacterial infection
Bacterial pneumonia	– Infiltrates in mycobacterial infections persist longer and responds less well to treatment

Tips and Pitfalls

The disorder cannot be clearly distinguished from tuberculosis solely on the basis of morphologic findings on the radiograph.

Selected References

Erasmus JJ, McAdams HP, Farrell MA et al. Pulmonary nontuberculous mycobacterial infection: radiologic manifestations. Radiographics 1999; 19: 1487–1505

Glassroth J. Pulmonary disease due to nontuberculous mycobacteria. Chest 2008; 133: 243–251

Martinez S, McAdams HP, Batchu CS. The many faces of pulmonary nontuberculous mycobacterial infection. AJR Am J Roentgenol 2007; 189: 177–186

Definition

▶ **Epidemiology**
The most common pathogens in immunocompetent patients are influenza A and B viruses in adults and parainfluenza and respiratory syncytial viruses in children ● The most common pathogens in immunocompromised patients (AIDS, immunosuppression) are measles virus, cytomegalovirus, and herpes zoster and herpes simplex viruses.

▶ **Etiology, pathophysiology, pathogenesis**
Infection by inhaled viruses including those that do not normally colonize the lung ● Mixed inflammatory reaction (primarily lymphocytic) within the central and peripheral airways and pulmonary interstitium ● This leads to impaired gas exchange.

Imaging Signs

▶ **Modality of choice**
CT is preferable to plain radiography.

▶ **Radiographic findings**
Reticular streaky interstitial shadowing (unilateral or bilateral), often diffuse, occasionally confluent ● Cytomegalovirus pneumonia usually exhibits bilateral symmetric reticulonodular densities ● Hilar lymphadenopathy ● Bacterial superinfection produces an alveolar pattern of dense consolidations ● Pleural effusion is rare.

▶ **CT findings**
Affected parenchymal segments show focal or diffuse ground-glass opacification ● Bronchial walls appear widened and blurred due to inflammatory peribronchial edema ("tree-in-bud" sign) and bronchiectasis ● The interlobar septa are accentuated.

▶ **Pathognomonic findings on chest radiograph**
Focal or diffuse interstitial shadowing in a febrile patient.

Clinical Aspects

▶ **Typical presentation**
Cough, fever, and myalgia in the prodromal phase ● Dyspnea, tachypnea, and cyanosis in the pneumonic phase.

▶ **Therapeutic options**
Treatment is supportive ● Aciclovir for herpesvirus infection ● Ganciclovir for cytomegalovirus infection ● Antibiotics for bacterial superinfection.

▶ **Course and prognosis**
Course is variable ● Outcome depends on the virulence of the pathogen and the patient's immune status ● Immunocompetent patients recover completely within 3 weeks.

▶ **What does the clinician want to know?**
Diagnosis ● Differential diagnosis ● Complications.

Fig. 4.15 Viral pneumonia in a 17-year-old boy with acute febrile infection, beginning with obstructive bronchitis and progressing within hours to respiratory insufficiency. The plain chest radiograph and CT scan show homogeneous opacification of all lung fields with denser shadowing bilaterally in the posterobasal segments. Barotrauma due to artificial respiration with mediastinal and interstitial emphysema and pneumonia on the left side.

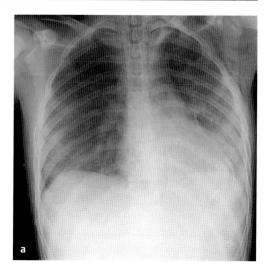

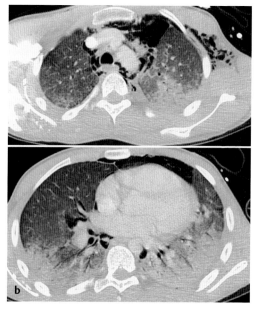

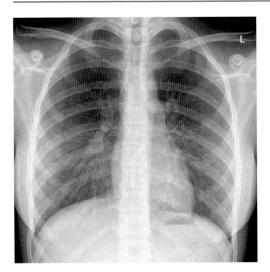

Fig. 4.16 Viral infection in a 24-year-old woman. The plain chest radiograph shows streaky bronchovascular shadowing in the right paracardiac and perihilar areas with slight opacification in the right lower lung field.

Differential Diagnosis

Pulmonary edema	– Symmetric densities and cranialization of vascular structures – Cardiomegaly – Pleural effusion
Pulmonary hemorrhage	– Hemoptysis and anemia – No lymphadenopathy – No signs of inflammation
Alveolar proteinosis	– Symmetric central densities ("bat's wing" sign) – Characteristic lavage findings – Chronicity

Tips and Pitfalls

Radiographic morphology does not provide reliable etiologic information.

Selected References

Müller NL et al. High-resolution CT findings of severe acute respiratory syndrome at presentation and after admission. AJR Am J Roentgenol 2004; 182: 39–44

Oikonomou A, Müller NL, Nantel S. Radiographic and high-resolution CT findings of influenza virus pneumonia in patients with hematologic malignancies. Am J Roentgenol 2003; 181: 507–511

Wong KT et al. Severe acute respiratory syndrome: radiographic appearances and pattern of progression in 138 patients. Radiology 2003; 228: 401–406

Definition

▶ **Epidemiology**
Cytomegalovirus is a ubiquitous DNA virus belong to the group of beta-herpesviruses • High prevalence worldwide (> 50%) with lifelong persistence • Infection usually goes unnoticed in immunocompetent people, but manifests itself clinically in immunocompromised patients (AIDS, transplantation).

▶ **Etiology, pathophysiology, pathogenesis**
Transmission occurs by contact, transfusion, or organ transplantation • Infection in immunocompromised patients occurs by reactivation (endogenous reinfection) or exogenous reinfection • Viral cytotoxicity causes parenchymal damage • Interstitial pneumonia • Diffuse alveolar damage.

Imaging Signs

▶ **Modality of choice**
Radiographs, CT.

▶ **Radiographs and CT**
Imaging findings cover a broad spectrum, depending on immunocompetence; findings may be nearly normal • Ground-glass opacities • Small nodular lesions • Consolidations • Changes are usually bilateral and diffuse.

▶ **Pathognomonic findings**
A bilateral ground-glass opacity in an at-risk patient is the finding most suggestive of infection.

Clinical Aspects

▶ **Typical presentation**
Depends on the patient's immune status • Fever • Unproductive cough • Dyspnea.

▶ **Therapeutic options**
Antiviral therapy (ganciclovir), also as prophylaxis.

▶ **Course and prognosis**
Mortality is about 5%.

▶ **What does the clinician want to know?**
Tentative diagnosis.

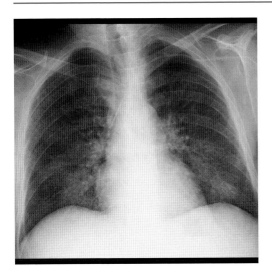

Fig. 4.17 Cytomegalovirus pneumonia. The radiograph shows finely nodular foci with a minimally dense ground-glass appearance are distributed over both lung fields. The perihilar and basal foci form larger confluent patterns. With their nearly symmetric distribution and concentration in the perihilar region, the findings resemble an edema.

Differential Diagnosis

Bacterial pneumonias	– Denser focal infiltrates
Mycotic pneumonias	– Slow-changing focal infiltrates
Varicella or herpes pneumonia	– Clinical aspects
	– Fulminant course
	– Extensive alveolar consolidations
Pneumocystis pneumonia	– Morphologically indistinguishable
Rejection or other complications of transplantation	– Morphologically indistinguishable
	– Timeframe for development of cytomegalovirus pneumonia is between 1 and 5 months after transplantation

Tips and Pitfalls

Indistinguishable from acute rejection of a lung transplant • In immunodeficiency due to other causes, findings are difficult to distinguish from *Pneumocystis jirovecii* pneumonia.

Selected References

Collins J et al. CT findings of pneumonia after lung transplantation. AJR Am J Roentgenol 2000; 175: 811–818

Horger M et al. [HRCT-Diagnostik der CMV-Pneumonie.] Fortschr Röntgenstr 2005; 177: 485–488 [In German]

Definition

▶ **Epidemiology**
With the exception of certain mycoses that are endemic to North America (blastomycosis, histoplasmosis, coccidiomycosis), these are opportunistic infections ● Infection occurs primarily in immunocompromised patients (transplantation, AIDS, chemotherapy) ● Fungi facultatively pathogenic in humans include *Cryptococcus neoformans*, *Candida*, and *Aspergillus* species.

▶ **Etiology, pathophysiology, pathogenesis**
– *Aspergillus* species: Usually *Aspergillus fumigatus* ● Infection may manifest itself in several forms: Invasive aspergillosis in severe immunodeficiency (leukocytes < 500/mm³, 80% vascular invasion, 15% airway invasion) ● Semi-invasive (chronic necrotizing) aspergillosis in low-grade immunodeficiency ● Allergic bronchopulmonary aspergillosis ● Saprophytic aspergilloma in chronic lung disease.
– *Candida* species: The most important is *Candida albicans* ● This species is part of the normal flora of the gastrointestinal tract and the skin ● Infection is via aspiration or hematogenously, usually in the setting of *Candida* sepsis with involvement of multiple organ systems.
– *Cryptococcus neoformans*: Found in pigeon excrement ● Airborne transmission ● Often involves the brain and meninges in addition to the lung.

Imaging Signs

▶ **Modality of choice**
CT is preferable to plain radiography.

▶ **Radiographs and CT**
– *Aspergillosis:* Invasive vascular aspergillosis produces segmental, lobar, or nodular shadowing with an initial halo; the "air crescent" sign is seen in resolving disease (after 2 weeks) ● Invasive airway aspergillosis produces a nonspecific picture comparable with bronchopneumonia ● In contrast, semi-invasive aspergillosis has a chronic course, producing a picture resembling tuberculosis, upper lobe infiltrate with cavitation ● Allergic bronchopulmonary aspergillosis ● Aspergilloma.
– *Candidiasis:* Unilocular or multilocular nodular focal infiltrates occurring primarily in the lower lobes with a more or less pronounced halo ● Interstitial micronodular or macronodular changes ● A miliary picture is possible, but rare (in endobronchial spread) ● Pleural effusion occurs in 25% of cases ● Cavitations and lymphadenopathy are rare.
– *Cryptococcosis:* Immunocompetent patients show peripheral nodular changes without cavitation ● Immunocompromised patients show variable changes: reticulonodular, miliary, or larger circumscribed foci (up to several centimeters) ● Cavitations, lymphadenopathy, and pleural effusion are rare (10–15% of cases).

▶ **Pathognomonic findings**
Multilocular focal infiltrates with or without cavitation and with a more or less pronounced halo are the findings most suggestive of pulmonary mycosis.

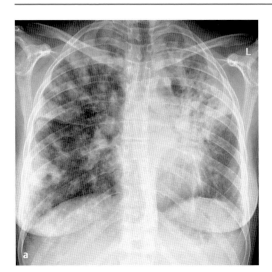

Fig. 4.18 Nocardiosis in a 32-year-old woman secondary to immunosuppressant therapy for vasculitis. The chest radiograph (**a**) shows bilateral, partially confluent round focal infiltrates. CT (**b**) reveals them as areas of liquefaction with mycetoma formation.

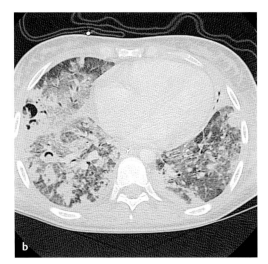

Clinical Aspects

▶ **Typical presentation**
Unspecific • Nonproductive cough • Shortness of breath • Chest pain • Occasionally fever.

Fig. 4.19 Fungal pneumonia in a 59-year-old man. The chest radiograph shows multiple ill-defined focal infiltrates 1.5 cm in diameter in both lungs. No liquefaction is visible. In conjunction with clinical findings (recurrent acute myeloid leukemia under treatment) the radiograph is suggestive of fungal pneumonia.

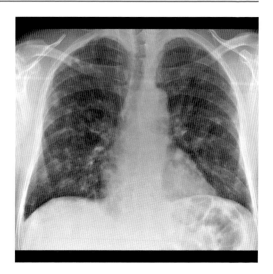

▶ **Confirmation of the diagnosis**
Definitive diagnosis requires a positive fungal culture from infected tissue or positive microscopic findings.

▶ **Therapeutic options**
Antimycotic therapy (amphotericin B, ketoconazole) ● Improvement of immunocompetence (for example with antiviral therapy in HIV infection).

▶ **Course and prognosis**
Depend on the underlying disorder and the patient's immunocompetence.

▶ **What does the clinician want to know?**
Confirmation of a tentative diagnosis ● Evaluation of the course.

Differential Diagnosis

Other opportunistic infections or pneumonias	– *Pneumocystis jirovecii* and cytomegalovirus infections – Show primarily interstitial, often edemalike, shadowing with ground-glass opacity
Postprimary tuberculosis, atypical mycobact. disease	– Radiographic morphology not clearly distinguishable from semi-invasive aspergillosis

Tips and Pitfalls

Can be misinterpreted as bacterial pneumonia ● Antibiotics will be ineffective.

Selected Reference

McAdams HP et al. Thoracic mycoses from endemic fungi/thoracic mycoses from opportunistic fungi: radiologic-pathologic correlation. Radiographics 1995; 15: 255–270, 271–286

Definition

▶ **Epidemiology**

Infection with *Aspergillus* spores (*Aspergillus fumigatus* in 80% of cases), a ubiquitous germ facultatively pathogenic in humans.

▶ **Etiology, pathophysiology, pathogenesis**

Descending colonization of tracheobronchial tree • Manifestation is variable, depending on immunocompetence:

- *Allergic bronchopulmonary aspergillosis:* Hypersensitivity reaction of the bronchial system and adjacent lung tissue in atopic patients with bronchial asthma or in cystic fibrosis.
- *Aspergilloma:* Colonization of preexisting cavities (tuberculous cavities, abscess).
- *Invasive pulmonary aspergillosis:* Opportunistic infection with granulomatous infiltrates, infarct pneumonia, and liquefaction in immunocompromised patients (acute myeloid leukemia, lymphoma, organ transplantation, underlying chronic wasting disease).
- Phenomena associated with aspergillosis: Asthma • Extrinsic allergic alveolitis • Eosinophilic pneumonia.

Imaging Signs

▶ **Modality of choice**

CT is greatly preferable to plain radiography.

▶ **Radiographic findings**

Initial imaging findings may be normal or discrete, in contrast to clinical findings • Later findings may include focal infiltrates or the picture of infarct pneumonia.

▶ **CT findings**

Solitary or multiple nodular opacities of varying size with a ground-glass peripheral zone (hemorrhagic "halo" sign) • Wedge-shaped subpleural infiltrates secondary to mycotic infarct • Confluent infiltrate resembling bronchopneumonia • Formation of a peripheral zone of lesser density and/or an "air crescent" sign indicates that healing has begun.

▶ **Pathognomonic findings**

Focal infiltrates with halo sign • "Air crescent" sign.

Clinical Aspects

▶ **Typical presentation**

Fever • Progressive dyspnea • Cough • Hemoptysis • Septic complications.

▶ **Therapeutic options**

Antimycotics.

▶ **Course and prognosis**

Variable • This depends on the underlying disorder.

▶ **What does the clinician want to know?**

Diagnosis and differential diagnosis.

Fig. 4.20 Aspergillosis in a 25-year-old woman with acute myeloid leukemia.

a, b The plain chest radiograph prior to treatment shows a homogeneous area of infiltrate resembling alveolar pneumonia. On CT it appears as a wedge-shaped lesion resembling an infarct.

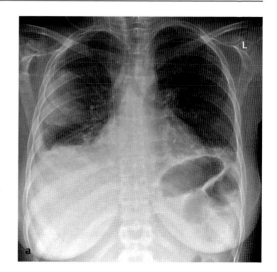

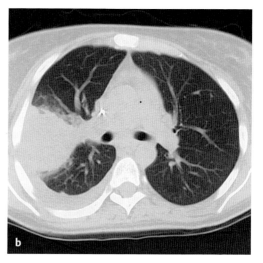

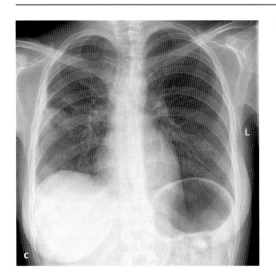

c, d The plain radiograph shows that the transradiancy has increased markedly following therapy and a broad "air crescent" has formed along the upper edge of the lesion. The CT scan shows the typical picture of a mycetoma.

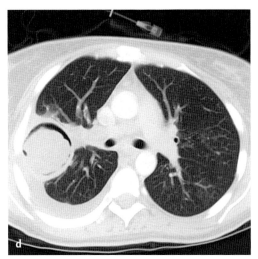

Differential Diagnosis

Halo sign	– General finding in pulmonary mycotic disease, rare in highly vascularized metastases or tumors, mycobacterial infections, cytomegalovirus or herpes pneumonia, and Wegener granulomatosis
Air crescent sign	– General finding in pulmonary mycotic disease, rare in necrotic tumors or bacterial pulmonary abscess
Bacterial pneumonia	– Hilar and/or mediastinal lymphadenopathy – Pleural effusion – Responds to antibiotics

Tips and Pitfalls

Can be misinterpreted as nonspecific pneumonic infiltrate.

Selected References

Althoff Souza C et al. Pulmonary invasive aspergillosis and candidiasis in immunocompromised patients: a comparative study of the high-resolution CT findings. J Thorac Imaging 2006; 21: 184–189

Franquet T et al. Spectrum of pulmonary aspergillosis: histologic, clinical, and radiologic findings. Radiographics 2001; 21: 825–837

Definition

▶ **Epidemiology**
Conglomerate of hyphae (*Aspergillus fumigatus*) and cell detritus in a preexisting cavity occurring secondary to a preexisting pulmonary disorder ● Prolonged antibiotic or steroid therapy ● Predilection for the male sex.

▶ **Etiology, pathophysiology, pathogenesis**
Fungal colonization of preexisting cavities (tuberculous cavities, abscess), descending along the tracheobronchial tree ● Locally destructive in immunocompromised patients (semi-invasive chronic necrotizing pulmonary aspergillosis).

Imaging Signs

▶ **Modality of choice**
CT is preferable to plain radiography.

▶ **Radiographic and CT findings**
Round focal lesion (1–5 cm) isodense to soft tissue, demarcated by a round or crescentic air gap (depending on patient positioning) surrounded by a ring of opacity ● Infiltrate with "air crescent" sign ● The fungus ball resembles a sponge on the CT scan due to air inclusions ● Usually occurs in the upper lobe or apical segment of the lower lobe (in tuberculous cavities).

▶ **Pathognomonic findings**
Mycetoma in a cavity ● "Air crescent" sign.

Clinical Aspects

▶ **Typical presentation**
Minimally symptomatic ● Often an incidental finding ● Hemoptysis occurs in 70% of cases (may be massive and life-threatening) ● Dyspnea, cough, and fever are usually symptomatic of the preexisting disorder.

▶ **Therapeutic options**
Antimycotics ● Intracavitary instillation may also be indicated ● Surgical management of hemoptysis.

▶ **Course and prognosis**
Variable ● This depends on the underlying disorder ● Prognosis is good for a stable clinical course; this does not apply to massive hemoptysis, which has a mortality rate of 5–10%.

▶ **What does the clinician want to know?**
Diagnosis and differential diagnosis.

Fig. 4.21 Aspergilloma (mycetoma) in a 65-year-old man. Both the plain chest radiograph and CT show typical ring shadows with central opacities bilaterally.

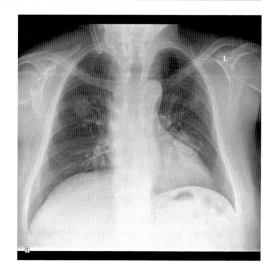

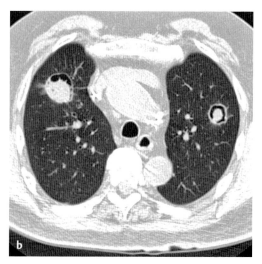

Differential Diagnosis

Other pulmonary mycosis or mycobacterial infection	– May be morphologically indistinguishable – Microbiology
Abscess-forming pneumonia or pulmonary abscess	– History – Course
Pulmonary laceration and/or hematoma	– History – Course
Nonsmall cell lung cancer	– Tumor constellation – History
Wegener granulomatosis	– Usually multilocular – No preexisting pulmonary pathology

Tips and Pitfalls

Rarely misinterpreted but possibly could be mistaken for a pulmonary abscess.

Selected References

Althoff Souza C et al. Pulmonary invasive aspergillosis and candidiasis in immunocompromised patients: a comparative study of the high-resolution CT findings. J Thorac Imaging 2006; 21: 184–189

Franquet T et al. Spectrum of pulmonary aspergillosis: histologic, clinical, and radiologic findings. Radiographics 2001; 21: 825–837

Definition

▶ **Epidemiology**
Opportunistic infection occurring in immunodeficiency due—in descending order—to AIDS, immunosuppressant therapy (transplant recipients, long-term steroid therapy), or congenital immune defect.

▶ **Etiology, pathophysiology, pathogenesis**
Infection by *Pneumocystis jirovecii* in the presence of a defect in cellular immunity (T-cell immune defect) ● This leads to interstitial pneumonia with foamy intraalveolar exudate ● Necrotizing granuloma and subpleural bullae occur in the presence of AIDS cysts.

Imaging Signs

▶ **Modality of choice**
Radiographs, CT.

▶ **Radiographic findings**
Perihilar or diffuse ground-glass opacity ● Secondary consolidation.

▶ **CT findings**
Bilateral areas of ground-glass opacification ● In association with septal thickening this produces a "crazy paving" pattern ● Upper lobe cysts occur in up to 30% of cases, creating a risk of pneumothorax ● No pleural effusion.

▶ **Pathognomonic findings**
Ground-glass opacification most pronounced in the perihilar region.

Clinical Aspects

▶ **Typical presentation**
AIDS patient (CD4 cells < 200/µL) ● Nonproductive cough ● Fever ● Dyspnea with the slightest exercise.

▶ **Therapeutic options**
Trimethoprim or pentamidine therapy ● In HIV infection, prophylaxis with pentamidine aerosol.

▶ **Course and prognosis**
Prognosis is good with prompt and adequate therapy.

▶ **What does the clinician want to know?**
Confirmation of a tentative diagnosis in at-risk patients.

Differential Diagnosis

Pulmonary edema (not cardiac)	– Acute onset – No fever – Slight pleural effusion
Cytomegalovirus pneumonia	– Often combined with *P. jirovecii* pneumonia (mixed infection)

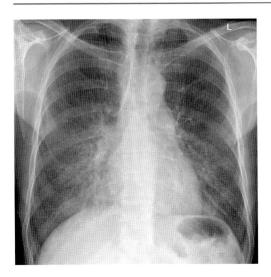

Fig. 4.22 *P. jirovecii* pneumonia in a 51-year-old man. The plain chest radiograph shows perihilar and paracardiac interstitial shadowing with masking of vascular structures, more marked on the right side.

Pulmonary hemorrhage	– Marked bilateral ground-glass opacification with areas of consolidation – Acute onset – Hemoptysis – Known predisposing underlying disease
Extrinsic allergic alveolitis	– Diffuse ground-glass opacity with centrilobular nodules – Subacute chronic course
Alveolar proteinosis	– "Crazy paving" pattern – Minimally symptomatic – Chronic course

Tips and Pitfalls

Discrete changes can lead to false-negative findings ● Initial progression of findings during treatment is consistent with fluid overload and must not be interpreted as worsening of the condition.

Selected References

Crans CA, Boiselle PM. Imaging features of Pneumocystis carinii pneumonia. Crit Rev Diagn Imaging 1999; 40: 251–284

Feldman C. Pneumonia associated with HIV infection. Curr Opin Infect Dis 2005; 18: 165–170

Definition

Idiopathic pulmonary fibrosis is classified by the American Thoracic Society (ATS) and European Respiratory Society (ERS) as an idiopathic interstitial pneumonia (chronic form of idiopathic interstitial pneumonia).

► **Epidemiology**
  Most common form of idiopathic interstitial pneumonia, accounting for about 50% of cases ● Occurs at age 40–50 years ● More common in men than in women.

► **Etiology, pathophysiology, pathogenesis**
  Inflammatory fibrotic disorder of the pulmonary parenchyma of uncertain etiology ● Areas of fibrotic changes in various stages alternating with normal parenchyma ● Nodular fibrosis and honeycomb cystic destruction.

Imaging Signs

► **Modality of choice**
  CT.

► **Radiographic findings**
  Reticular shadowing, primarily in the basal segments.

► **CT findings**
  Reticular shadowing ● Honeycombing ● Traction bronchiectasis ● Focal ground-glass opacities ● Disorganization of pulmonary architecture ● Predilection for the peripheral, basal, and subpleural regions ● Apicobasal gradient.

► **Pathognomonic findings**
  CT findings in the context of corresponding clinical data are diagnostic (sensitivity is about 50%, specificity > 90%, positive predictive value > 90%); biopsy is not required.

Clinical Aspects

► **Typical presentation**
  Initially insidious but progressive respiratory distress over > 6 months ● Nonproductive cough ● Clubbed fingers (occurs in up to 50% of cases).

► **Therapeutic options**
  Responds to steroids only in combination with ciclosporin ● Lung transplant.

► **Course and prognosis**
  Prognosis is not favorable ● Median survival time after diagnosis is 2.5–3.5 years.

► **What does the clinician want to know?**
  Confirmation of the diagnosis ● Course ● Complications (other opportunistic infections, *Pneumocystis jirovecii* pneumonia).

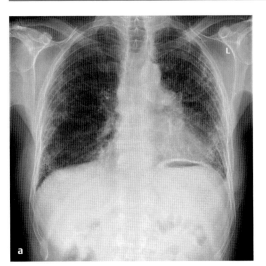

Fig. 5.1 Idiopathic pulmonary fibrosis.

a The plain chest radiograph shows extensive, primarily reticular and honeycomb interstitial changes.

b CT shows primarily basal and peripheral subpleural interstitial honeycombing. The trabeculation of the pleural boundaries (arrow), bronchiectasis resembling a string of pearls (open arrow), ectasia of the trachea and main bronchi (∗) are further signs.

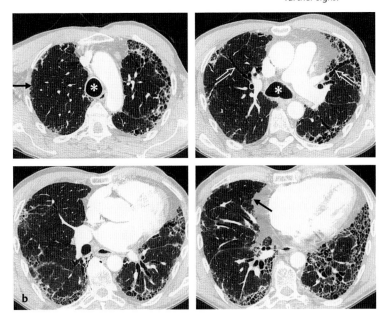

Differential Diagnosis

Other forms of idiopathic interstitial pneumonia	– Micronodules are inconsistent with idiopathic pulmonary fibrosis – Extensive ground-glass opacities – Consolidations – Peribronchovascular distribution
Secondary interstitial pneumonia	– Pulmonary involvement in collagen diseases, vasculitis, drug reactions, or inhaled noxious agents
Cryptogenic organizing pneumonia	– Cryptogenic organizing pneumonia with a reticular pattern can be difficult to distinguish from diffuse pulmonary fibrosis
Extrinsic allergic alveolitis (hypersensitivity pneumonitis)	– Exposure to allergens – Mosaic pattern

Tips and Pitfalls

Radiographic findings are often suggestive and permit a diagnosis in about 70% of cases.

Selected References

American Thoracic Society/European Respiratory Society. International multidisciplinary consensus classification of the idiopathic interstitial pneumonias. Am J Respir Crit Care Med 2002; 165: 277–304

Kim DS, Collard HR, King TE. Classification and natural history of the idiopathic interstitial pneumonias. Proc Am Thor Soc 2006; 3: 285–292

Müller-Lang C et al. [Idiopathische interstitielle Pneumonien.] Radiologe 2007; 47: 384–392 [In German]

Wittram C, Mark EJ, McLoud TC. CT-histologic correlation of the ATS/ERS 2002 classification of idiopathic interstitial pneumonias. Radiographics 2003; 23: 1057–1071

Definition

Cryptogenic organizing pneumonia is classified by the ATS and ERS as an idiopathic interstitial pneumonia (subacute form of idiopathic interstitial pneumonia) • Formerly referred to as bronchiolitis obliterans.

▶ **Epidemiology**
Idiopathic cryptogenic organizing pneumonia is a rare form of idiopathic interstitial pneumonia, accounting for about 10% of cases • Occurs at age 40–50 years • No sex predilection • More common in smokers than in nonsmokers.

▶ **Etiology, pathophysiology, pathogenesis**
Rare in its idiopathic form; more common secondary to collagen diseases and infectious or drug-induced pulmonary disorders • Polypoid granulomatous inflammation of the respiratory bronchioles and alveoli without disorganization of the pulmonary architecture.

Imaging Signs

▶ **Modality of choice**
CT.

▶ **Radiographic findings**
Unilateral or bilateral nodular opacities • Resembles pneumonia.

▶ **CT**
Bilateral focal non-segmental consolidations in the subpleural or peribronchial regions (>80% of cases) • Tendency to migrate • An air bronchogram is common • Perifocal ground-glass opacity (in 60% of cases) • Peribronchiolar centrilobular round focal lesions < 10 mm with irregular borders in up to 50% of cases.

▶ **Pathognomonic findings**
Focal areas of consolidation with air bronchogram and associated ground-glass opacification in the subpleural or peribronchial region • Findings are unchanged or progressive for weeks despite antibiotics.

Clinical Aspects

▶ **Typical presentation**
Subacute onset over a period of up to 3 months • Nonproductive cough • Subfebrile temperatures • Often a lower airway infection is initially suspected • Restrictive pulmonary dysfunction.

▶ **Confirmation of the diagnosis**
Biopsy.

▶ **Therapeutic options**
Inhalational or systemic steroids.

▶ **Course and prognosis**
Prognosis is good with steroid therapy.

▶ **What does the clinician want to know?**
Diagnosis • Course under therapy.

Fig. 5.2 Cryptogenic organizing pneumonia in a 67-year-old woman.

a The plain chest radiograph shows isolated moderately sharply demarcated focal densities bilaterally but primarily on the right side. The right hilar bronchovascular bundles appear slightly thickened.

b CT shows the focal lesions as homogeneous areas of consolidation with isolated excursions but otherwise without any reaction in the adjacent tissue.

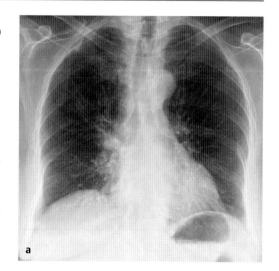

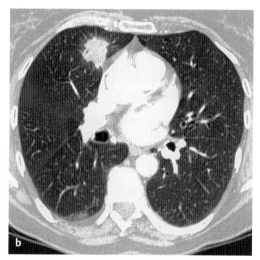

Differential Diagnosis

Bronchioalveolar carcinoma	– History – Lung biopsy
Pneumonia or bronchopneumonia	– Usually unilateral and unilocular – Responds to antibiotics
Eosinophilic pneumonia	– Predilection for the upper lobes – Blood eosinophilia
Sarcoidosis	– Predilection for the bronchovascular bundle – Lymphadenopathy
Lymphoma	– Known underlying disease – Extrathoracic involvement
Reaction as in bronchiolitis obliterans	– Occurs in collagen diseases – Drug reaction – Toxic damage from inhaled agent – Sequela of aspiration – Postinfectious

Tips and Pitfalls

Can be misinterpreted as pneumonia.

Selected References

American Thoracic Society/European Respiratory Society. International multidisciplinary consensus classification of the idiopathic interstitial pneumonias. Am J Respir Crit Care Med 2002; 165: 277–304

Bouchardy LM et al. CT findings in bronchiolitis obliterans organizing pneumonia (BOOP) with radiographic, clinical, and histologic correlation. JCAT 1993; 17: 352–357

Hartmann TE et al. CT of bronchial and bronchiolar diseases. Radiographics 1994; 14: 991–1003

Kim DS, Collard HR, King TE. Classification and natural history of the idiopathic interstitial pneumonias. Proc Am Thor Soc 2006; 3: 285–292

Lynch DA et al. Idiopathic interstitial pneumonias. CT features. Radiology 2005; 236: 10–21

Müller-Lang C et al. [Idiopathische interstitielle Pneumonien.] Radiologe 2007; 47: 384–392 [In German]

Wittram C, Mark EJ, McLoud TC. CT-histologic correlation of the ATS/ERS 2002 classification of idiopathic interstitial pneumonias. Radiographics 2003; 23: 1057–1071

Definition

Desquamative interstitial pneumonia is classified by the ATS and ERS as an idiopathic interstitial pneumonia (subacute form of idiopathic interstitial pneumonia).

▶ **Epidemiology**

Along with respiratory bronchiolitis with interstitial lung disease, this is the third most common form of idiopathic interstitial pneumonia, accounting for about 13% of all cases ● Occurs almost exclusively in smokers (> 90% of cases) ● Occurs at age 30–50 years ● Twice as common in men than in women.

▶ **Etiology, pathophysiology, pathogenesis**

Lung damage from chronic smoking includes bronchiolitis, which leads to respiratory bronchiolitis with interstitial lung disease, which in turn leads to desquamative interstitial pneumonia (idiopathic interstitial pneumonia) ● Characterized by accumulation of macrophages around the respiratory bronchioles and slight interstitial fibrosis.

Imaging Signs

▶ **Modality of choice**

CT.

▶ **Radiographic findings**

Findings are normal in about 20% of cases ● There may be discrete patchy densities with a finely reticular striped pattern, more pronounced in the basal region (lower lung fields).

▶ **CT findings**

A variable distribution of ground-glass opacities is a nearly universal finding ● Reticular basal and subpleural reticular shadowing ● Isolated small cysts (indicative of traction bronchiolectasis) ● Pulmonary architecture is preserved ● No location predilection: Basal and subpleural (60% of cases), nodular (25%), disseminated, or diffuse (15%).

▶ **Pathognomonic findings**

Smoker with diffuse ground-glass opacification on CT.

Clinical Aspects

▶ **Typical presentation**

Subacute onset over a period of up to 3 months with dyspnea and nonproductive cough ● Clubbed fingers (50% of cases) ● History of smoking.

▶ **Confirmation of the diagnosis**

In patients requiring treatment, the diagnosis is confirmed by biopsy.

▶ **Therapeutic options**

Tobacco abstinence ● Steroids.

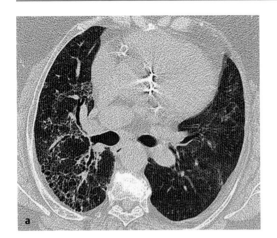

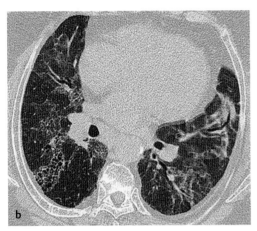

Fig. 5.3 Desquamative interstitial pneumonia in a 56-year-old man. CT shows varying regional changes, some in the form of reticular densities with isolated cysts, some as focal ground-glass opacities.

▶ **Course and prognosis**

Prognosis is good with tobacco abstinence and steroids where indicated • 10-year survival rate is about 70%.

▶ **What does the clinician want to know?**

Confirmation of the tentative diagnosis • Extent of changes.

Differential Diagnosis

Respiratory bronchiolitis with interstitial lung disease	– More nodular areas of ground-glass opacification – Low-density centrilobular nodules
Extrinsic allergic alveolitis	– Nonsmoker – Exposure to allergens – Mosaic pattern
Nonspecific interstitial pneumonitis	– Ambiguous radiographic morphology – Indistinguishable – Most often confused with this disorder
Sarcoidosis	– Predilection for the bronchovascular bundle – Lymphadenopathy
Idiopathic pulmonary fibrosis	– Fibrosis with honeycombing, especially in the basal subpleural region – Disorganization of pulmonary architecture
Lymphocytic interstitial pneumonitis	– Ambiguous or identical radiographic morphology – Associated with collagen diseases, immune defects, and Sjögren syndrome
Secondary interstitial pneumonia	– Pulmonary involvement in collagen diseases, vasculitis, drug reactions, or inhaled noxious agents
Pneumocystis jirovecii pneumonia	– History – HIV infection

Tips and Pitfalls

Most often confused with nonspecific interstitial pneumonitis.

Selected References

Desai SR, Ryan SM, Colby TV. Smoking-related interstitial lung diseases: histological and imaging perspectives. Clin Radiol 2003; 58: 259–68

Kim DS, Collard HR, King TE. Classification and natural history of the idiopathic interstitial pneumonias. Proc Am Thor Soc 2006; 3: 285–292

Lynch DA et al. Idiopathic interstitial pneumonias: CT features. Radiology 2005; 236: 10–21

Wittram C, Mark EJ, McLoud TC. CT-histologic correlation of the ATS/ERS 2002 classification of idiopathic interstitial pneumonias. Radiographics 2003; 23: 1057–1071

Definition

Respiratory bronchiolitis with interstitial lung disease is classified by the ATS and ERS as an idiopathic interstitial pneumonia (chronic form of idiopathic interstitial pneumonia).

▶ **Epidemiology**

Along with desquamative interstitial pneumonia, this is the third most common form of idiopathic interstitial pneumonia, accounting for about 13% of cases • Occurs at age 30–40 years • Twice as common in men than in women • Occurs almost exclusively in smokers.

▶ **Etiology, pathophysiology, pathogenesis**

Bronchiolocentric distribution of alveolar macrophages accompanied by slight interstitial fibrosis.

Imaging Signs

▶ **Modality of choice**

CT.

▶ **Radiographic findings**

Findings are normal in about 20% of cases and otherwise nonspecific • Bronchial walls may appear more prominent (75% of cases) • Nodular ground-glass opacities (60%).

▶ **CT findings**

Findings are disseminated or primarily in the upper lobes. They include low-density centrilobular nodules (airspace nodules, ground-glass nodules) • Ground-glass opacities • Bronchial wall thickening • Centrilobular emphysema, often but not always located in the apical segments.

▶ **Pathognomonic findings**

Low-density centrilobular nodules.

Clinical Aspects

▶ **Typical presentation**

Minimally symptomatic • Slowly progressive dyspnea with dry cough in smokers • Severity of the symptoms depends largely on the associated emphysema • Bronchoalveolar lavage findings are nonspecific.

▶ **Therapeutic options**

Tobacco abstinence • Steroids where indicated.

▶ **Course and prognosis**

Prognosis is good and changes are partially reversible with tobacco abstinence.

Fig. 5.4 Respiratory bronchiolitis with interstitial lung disease in a 42-year-old woman smoker. CT shows disseminated ill-defined low-density centrilobular nodules (ground-glass nodules). The bronchial walls do not appear more prominent.

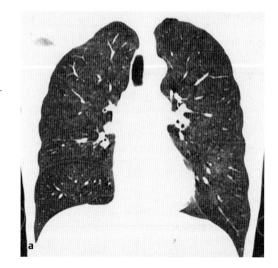

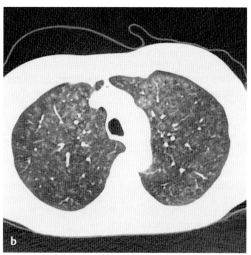

Differential Diagnosis

Desquamative interstitial pneumonia	– More diffuse ground-glass opacities – No centrilobular nodules
Extrinsic allergic alveolitis	– No centrilobular nodules – Nonsmoker – Exposure to allergens
Langerhans cell histiocytosis	– Micronodules are denser and more disseminated, with some liquefaction (cysts)

Selected References

American Thoracic Society/European Respiratory Society. International multidisciplinary consensus classification of the idiopathic interstitial pneumonias. Am J Respir Crit Care Med 2002; 165: 277–304

Kim DS, Collard HR, King TE. Classification and natural history of the idiopathic interstitial pneumonias. Proc Am Thor Soc 2006; 3: 285–292

Müller-Lang C et al. [Idiopathische interstitielle Pneumonien.] Radiologe 2007; 47: 384–392 [In German]

Wittram C, Mark EJ, McLoud TC. CT-histologic correlation of the ATS/ERS 2002 classification of idiopathic interstitial pneumonias. Radiographics 2003; 23: 1057–1071

Idiopathic Interstitial Pneumonia

Definition
....

Nonspecific interstitial pneumonitis is classified by the ATS and ERS as an idiopathic interstitial pneumonia (chronic form of idiopathic interstitial pneumonia). However, it is regarded as a "provisional diagnosis" because of unresolved issues.

▶ **Epidemiology**
Second most common form of idiopathic interstitial pneumonia, accounting for about 25% of cases • Occurs at age 30–40 years • No sex predilection • Unrelated to smoking • Also occurs in collagen vascular diseases.

▶ **Etiology, pathophysiology, pathogenesis**
Inflammatory fibrotic disorder of the pulmonary interstitium of uncertain etiology • Spatially and temporally homogeneous changes • The broad range of histologic changes can be categorized into one of two subtypes: cellular and fibrotic.

Imaging Signs
....

▶ **Modality of choice**
CT.

▶ **Radiographic findings**
Broad range of changes; nodular parenchymal changes occur most often.

▶ **CT findings**
Broad range of findings: Diffuse or nodular ground-glass opacities • Irregular linear or reticular shadowing • Micronodules • Bronchiectasis and bronchiolectasis • At most minimal honeycombing • Symmetric with predilection for the peripheral, basal, and subpleural regions • No apicobasal gradient.

▶ **Pathognomonic findings**
There is no pathognomonic constellation of findings • The initial diagnosis is correct in only 10% of cases • Most often confused with desquamative interstitial pneumonia • Biopsy is invariably indicated to confirm a tentative clinical and radiologic diagnosis.

Clinical Aspects
....

▶ **Typical presentation**
There is no distinctive clinical picture as such: Initially insidious but progressive dyspnea with nonproductive cough as in idiopathic pulmonary fibrosis, although not as severe • Fatigue • Weight loss • The diagnosis of nonspecific interstitial pneumonitis can usually be made only by observing the course of the disorder and excluding secondary forms (collagen diseases, extrinsic allergic alveolitis, drug reaction).

▶ **Confirmation of the diagnosis**
In patients requiring treatment, the diagnosis is confirmed by biopsy.

▶ **Therapeutic options**
Steroids.

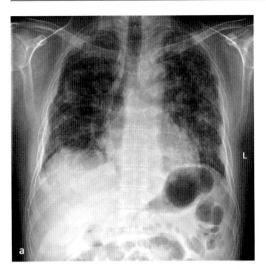

Fig. 5.5 Nonspecific interstitial pneumonitis in a 42-year-old man.

a The plain chest radiograph shows disseminated nodular parenchymal opacities over both lungs accompanied by reticular shadowing not primarily limited to the basal segments.

b Findings on CT include severe bronchiectasis and bronchiolectasis. Extensive pleural involvement.

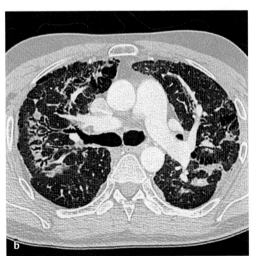

▶ **Course and prognosis**

Prognosis is more favorable than with idiopathic interstitial pneumonia ● Life expectancy is minimally reduced with the cellular subtype, moderately reduced with the fibrotic subtype (median survival > 10 years and < 10 years, respectively).

▶ **What does the clinician want to know?**

Differential diagnosis ● Activity of the disease ● Course.

Differential Diagnosis

Desquamative interstitial pneumonia	– Ambiguous radiographic morphology – Indistinguishable – Most often confused with this disorder
Idiopathic pulmonary fibrosis	– Hardly any ground-glass opacities or consolidations
Cryptogenic organizing pneumonia	– Subpleural and peribronchial focal areas of consolidation with an air bronchogram
Secondary interstitial pneumonia	– Pulmonary involvement in collagen diseases, vasculitis – Drug reactions or inhaled noxious agents
Alveolar proteinosis	– "Crazy paving" pattern interspersed with areas of normal parenchyma
Extrinsic allergic alveolitis (hypersensitivity pneumonitis)	– Exposure to allergens – Mosaic pattern

Tips and Pitfalls

Often confused with desquamative interstitial pneumonia.

Selected References

America Thoracic Society/European Respiratory Society. International multidisciplinary consensus classification of the idiopathic interstitial pneumonias. Am J Respir Crit Care Med 2002; 165: 277–304

Kim DS, Collard HR, King TE. Classification and natural history of the idiopathic interstitial pneumonias. Proc Am Thor Soc 2006; 3: 285–292

Müller-Lang C et al. [Idiopathische interstitielle Pneumonien.] Radiologe 2007; 47: 384–392 [In German]

Wittram C, Mark EJ, McLoud TC. CT-histologic correlation of the ATS/ERS 2002 classification of idiopathic interstitial pneumonias. Radiographics 2003; 23: 1057–1071

Definition

Lymphocytic interstitial pneumonitis is classified by the ATS and ERS as an idiopathic interstitial pneumonia (chronic form of idiopathic interstitial pneumonia) • Some authors classify it as a MALT lymphoma.

▶ **Epidemiology**
Very rare form of idiopathic interstitial pneumonia (< 2 % of cases) • Affects adults of all age groups • More common in women than in men • Often associated with autoimmune disorders or immunosuppressive or infectious disease (HIV, Epstein–Barr virus, *Pneumocystis jirovecii*).

▶ **Etiology, pathophysiology, pathogenesis**
Infiltration of the alveolar septa by lymphocytes, plasma cells, and macrophages.

Imaging Signs

▶ **Modality of choice**
CT.

▶ **Radiographic findings**
Reticulonodular shadowing.

▶ **CT findings**
Diffuse or primarily basal ground-glass opacities • Centrilobular and subpleural nodules • Thin-walled cysts of varying size.

▶ **Pathognomonic findings**
Ground-glass opacity with thin-walled cysts.

Clinical Aspects

▶ **Typical presentation**
Slow onset (> 12 months) with gradually increasing shortness of breath and cough • In secondary forms the symptoms of the underlying disorder predominate.

▶ **Confirmation of the diagnosis**
By biopsy • As the disorder is rare, secondary forms of interstitial pneumonia (collagen diseases, autoimmune disorders, primary sclerosing cholangitis, myasthenia, Hashimoto disease) should be excluded.

▶ **Therapeutic options**
Steroids.

▶ **Course and prognosis**
Prognosis is favorable • In rare cases can progress to malignant lymphoma.

▶ **What does the clinician want to know?**
Differential diagnosis • Activity of the disease.

Fig. 5.6 Lymphocytic interstitial pneumonitis in a 44-year-old woman.
a The plain chest radiograph shows only discrete reticulonodular shadowing.

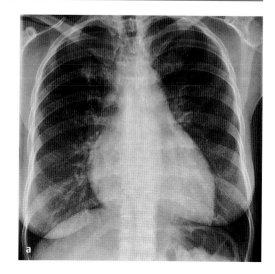

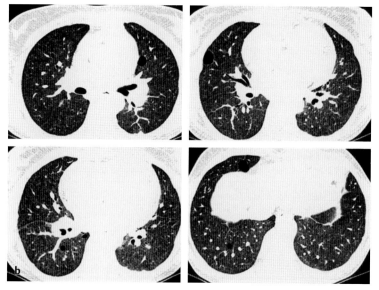

b CT findings predominantly include generalized ground-glass opacification and isolated thin-walled cysts.

Differential Diagnosis

Nonspecific interstitial pneumonitis	– Bronchovascular ground-glass opacities
Extrinsic allergic alveolitis	– No cystic changes
	– Exposure to allergens
Disorders with thin-walled cysts	– Langerhans cell histiocytosis
	– Lymphangioleiomyomatosis
	– Centrilobular emphysema
	– Laryngeal papillomatosis

Tips and Pitfalls

Nonspecific findings in a rare disorder may lead to incorrect diagnosis.

Selected References

American Thoracic Society/European Respiratory Society. International multidisciplinary consensus classification of the idiopathic interstitial pneumonias. Am J Respir Crit Care Med 2002; 165: 277–304

Nicholson AG. Lymphocytic interstitial pneumonia and other lymphoproliferative disorders in the lung. Semin Resp Crit Care Med 2001; 22: 409–422

Wittram C, Mark EJ, McLoud TC. CT-histologic correlation of the ATS/ERS 2002 classification of idiopathic interstitial pneumonias. Radiographics 2003; 23: 1057–1071

Definition

Generalized inflammatory joint disorder of uncertain etiology.

▶ **Epidemiology**
Most common collagen vascular disease • Extraarticular manifestations are rare • More common in men than women • Rarely occurs before joint symptoms • Occurs in middle age.

▶ **Etiology, pathophysiology, pathogenesis**
Etiology is unclear • Pleuropulmonary manifestations include pleural involvement and, less pronounced, fibrosing alveolitis, rheumatoid nodules, airway changes (bronchitis, bronchiolitis, bronchiectasis).

Imaging Signs

▶ **Modality of choice**
CT.

▶ **Radiographic findings**
Low sensitivity • Severe cases show predominantly basal reticulonodular shadowing and linear, nonseptal opacities • Honeycombing • Pleuritis (pleural effusion) • Rheumatoid nodules (< 5% of cases).

▶ **CT findings**
Pathologic findings are visualized in about 30% of cases.
  – *Pleural findings (most common):* Include slight pleural effusion • Pleural thickening.
  – *Parenchymal findings (predominantly basal and subpleural):* Include finely to coarsely reticular and nodular opacities with honeycombing, similar to idiopathic pulmonary fibrosis or nonspecific interstitial pneumonitis • Ground-glass opacities • Rheumatoid nodules (solitary or multiple, peripheral, sharply demarcated, 50% showing cavitation, rarely calcified).
  – *Airway findings:* Include bronchiolitis • Bronchiectasis.

▶ **Pathognomonic findings**
Coarsely reticular and nodular interstitial changes in combination with joint symptoms.

Clinical Aspects

▶ **Typical presentation**
Presentation is variable; patients may be asymptomatic • Dyspnea with nonproductive cough • Pleuritis • Lung function is restricted with impaired diffusion capacity and reduced vital capacity • Positive rheumatoid factor in 80% of cases • Pleural exudate is high in protein and low in glucose with a high level of lactate dehydrogenase and low pH and contains lymphocytic, neutrophilic, and eosinophilic cells.

▶ **Therapeutic options**
Anti-inflammatory treatment of the underlying disorder (anti-inflammatory agents, steroids, TNF-α blockers, immunosuppressives).

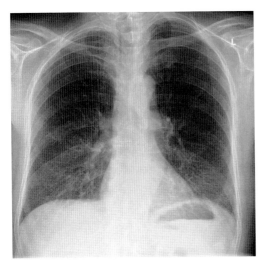

Fig. 6.1 Plain chest radiograph of a 70-year-old man with a long history of rheumatoid arthritis. Relatively nonspecific bilateral basal finely reticular streaky shadowing consistent with pulmonary interstitial changes.

▶ **Course and prognosis**
Depend on the underlying disorder.
▶ **What does the clinician want to know?**
Characterize and ascertain the extent of findings.

Differential Diagnosis

Idiopathic pulmonary fibrosis	– Ambiguous radiographic morphology
	– No pleural changes
	– No rheumatoid nodules
	– No joint pathology
Scleroderma	– Ambiguous radiographic morphology
	– Esophageal dilation
	– No joint pathology
Asbestosis	– Ambiguous radiographic morphology
	– Pleural plaques
	– History of occupational exposure

Tips and Pitfalls

In the presence of a known underlying disorder, the diagnosis is straightforward •
However, the findings themselves are nonspecific • Focal lesions require histologic evaluation.

Fig. 6.2 Rheumatoid nodules in a 70-year-old woman.

a The plain chest radiograph shows bilateral focal lesions, the largest of which occur in the left laterobasal pleural region.

b Findings on CT include isolated eccentric cavities and bronchiectatic changes.

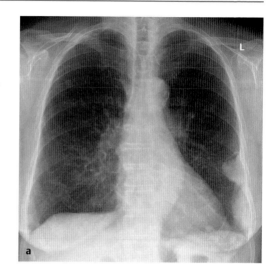

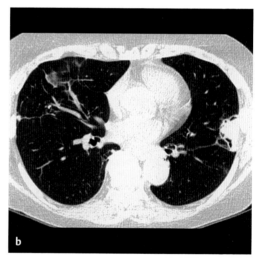

Selected References

Biederer J et al. Correlation between HRCT findings, pulmonary function tests and bronchoalveolar lavage cytology in interstitial lung disease associated with rheumatoid arthritis. Eur Radiol 2004; 14: 272–280

Remy-Jardin M et al. Lung changes in rheumatoid arthritis: CT findings. Radiology 1994; 193: 375–382

Definition

▶ **Epidemiology**
Systemic autoimmune disorder, a member of the group of collagen diseases.

▶ **Etiology, pathophysiology, pathogenesis**
Antinuclear antibodies are present in 95% of cases • Genetic disposition • 90% of patients are women • Pleuropulmonary involvement in about 50% of cases, usually in the form of pleural effusions, less often as acute lupus pneumonitis with damage to the alveolar-capillary membrane and alveolar hemorrhages • Pulmonary fibrosis rarely develops.

Imaging Signs

▶ **Modality of choice**
CT is preferable to plain radiography.

▶ **Radiographic and CT findings**
Pleuritis or pleural effusion in 70% of cases, pericardial effusion in 35% (usually slight and bilateral) • Lupus pneumonitis in 5% with nodular consolidations, ground-glass opacities, alveolar hemorrhages, predominantly basal • "Shrinking lung" syndrome: increasing volume loss without significant parenchymal changes (from diaphragmatic dysfunction or pleuritis) • Fibrosis, thickening of the bronchial wall, or bronchiectasis are rare • *Note:* Pneumonia is common in immunosuppression (whether pathologic or drug-induced).

▶ **Pathognomonic findings**
There are no pathognomonic findings. Pleural and pulmonary changes tend to be nonspecific.

Clinical Aspects

▶ **Typical presentation**
Presence of at least four of the following symptoms is diagnostic: butterfly erythema, discoid lupus, photosensitivity, oral ulcerations, arthritis, serositis, renal involvement, CNS involvement, antinuclear antibodies • With pulmonary involvement, symptoms include fever, dyspnea, cough, chest pain, and hemoptysis.

▶ **Therapeutic options**
Immunosuppressives.

▶ **Course and prognosis**
Depend on the organs involved.

Fig. 6.3

a Pleuritis with systemic lupus erythematosus. The plain chest radiograph of a patient with reduced depth of inspiration shows a left pleural effusion with strips of dystelectasis on the right.

b, c The CT scans show pericardial involvement in addition to the pleural effusion but no interstitial or parenchymal changes.

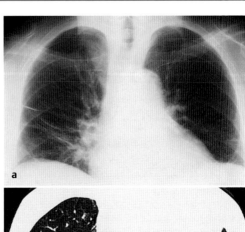

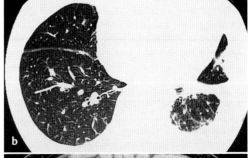

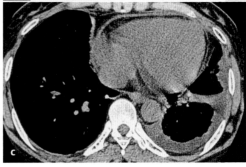

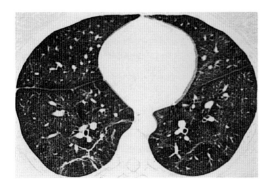

Fig. 6.4 CT in systemic lupus erythematosus showing discrete interstitial changes resembling ground-glass opacity.

Differential Diagnosis

Other collagen diseases	– Clinical findings are crucial to the diagnosis – Morphologic findings on the radiograph are usually ambiguous
Idiopathic interstitial pneumonia	– Pulmonary changes are most important and are crucial to the diagnosis
Pneumonia	– In systemic lupus erythematosus there is usually other pulmonary pathology with pleural involvement, pulmonary hemorrhage, and interstitial changes

Tips and Pitfalls

Consolidation can be misinterpreted and pneumonitis confused with pneumonia •
The "shrinking lung" syndrome can be overlooked in the absence of parenchymal changes.

Selected References

Fenlon HM et al. High-resolution chest CT in systemic lupus erythematosus. AJR Am J Roentgenol 1996; 166: 301–307

Kim JS et al. Thoracic involvement of systemic lupus erythematosus: clinical, pathologic, and radiologic findings. JCAT 2000; 24: 9–18

Lalani TA et al. Imaging findings in systemic lupus erythematosus. Radiographics 2004; 24: 1069–1086

Definition

▶ **Epidemiology**
A distinction is made between primary Sjögren syndrome (solitary occurrence) and secondary Sjögren syndrome (in association with other collagen vascular diseases, usually rheumatoid arthritis).

▶ **Etiology, pathophysiology, pathogenesis**
Usually manifests itself between the ages of 40 and 70 years ● More common in women than men ● Increase in antinuclear and anticytoplasmic antibodies ● Associated in 6% of cases with other collagen vascular diseases and with lymphomas ● Internal organs (such as the lungs) may be involved.

Imaging Signs

▶ **Modality of choice**
CT is preferable to plain radiography.

▶ **Radiographic and CT findings**
Pathologic findings in up to 30% of patients include reticular or reticulonodular shadowing ● Ground-glass opacities ● Bronchiectasis, usually predominantly basal ● Multiple pulmonary cysts (lymphocytic interstitial pneumonitis) ● Pleuritis with effusion.

▶ **Pathognomonic findings**
Cystic changes (lymphocytic interstitial pneumonitis) in an otherwise normal lung are relatively characteristic. The pulmonary pathology is otherwise nonspecific.

Clinical Aspects

▶ **Typical presentation**
Triad of xerostomia, keratoconjunctivitis sicca, and swelling of the parotid glands.

▶ **Therapeutic options**
No specific therapy is available ● Immunosuppression with steroids ● Symptomatic treatment of xerostomia and keratoconjunctivitis sicca.

▶ **Course and prognosis**
Depend on the associated disorders such as systemic lupus erythematosus or lymphoma.

Differential Diagnosis

Other rheumatic disorders
– Differential diagnosis is usually not possible solely on the basis of radiographic findings
– The nonspecific pulmonary changes occur in many disorders
– Clinical findings are crucial to the diagnosis

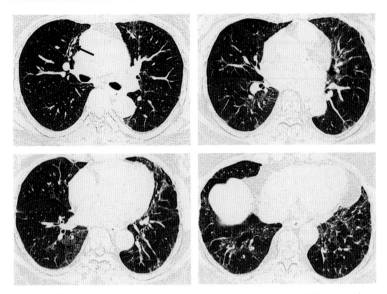

Fig. 6.5 Sjögren syndrome in a 64-year-old woman. The cross-sectional CT images show mostly coarser reticular changes primarily in the basal lung segments next to circumscribed areas of fine ground-glass opacification. Early bronchiectatic changes are seen (arrow).

Tips and Pitfalls

Subtle pulmonary pathology is often overlooked on radiographs.

Selected References

Franquet T et al. Primary Sjögren's syndrome and associated lung disease: CT findings in 50 patients. AJR Am J Roentgenol 1997; 169: 655–658

Lohrmann C et al. High-resolution CT imaging of the lung for patients with primary Sjogren's syndrome. Eur J Radiol 2004; 52: 137–143

Definition

▶ **Epidemiology**
Generalized connective tissue disorder, classified as a collagen disease • Peak occurrence is between the ages of 30 and 50 years • Women are affected three times as often as men.

▶ **Etiology, pathophysiology, pathogenesis**
Autoimmune disorder with connective tissue changes and vasculitis • Antinuclear antibodies • Skin changes • Raynaud phenomenon • Musculoskeletal and visceral manifestations (gastrointestinal tract, lung, heart, kidneys) • Pulmonary involvement occurs in about 75% of cases (associated with antitopoisomerase I antibodies) • Morphologic findings include fibrosing alveolitis, intimal proliferation, and medial hypertrophy of the small vessels.

Imaging Signs

▶ **Modality of choice**
CT is preferable to plain radiography.

▶ **Radiographic findings**
Predominantly basal reticulonodular shadowing • Esophageal dilatation.

▶ **CT findings**
Interlobular and intralobular finely reticular and/or reticulonodular interstitial shadowing (including ground-glass opacities and consolidations), primarily in the basal and subpleural regions • The reticulation becomes increasingly coarse over time, with traction bronchiolectasis and honeycombing • Pleural pathology or effusion occurs in 30% of cases • Esophageal dilatation occurs in 40–80% • Mediastinal lymphadenopathy occurs in 60%.

▶ **Pathognomonic findings**
Fibrotic interstitial changes predominantly in the basal and subpleural regions • Esophageal dilatation.

Clinical Aspects

▶ **Typical presentation**
Raynaud disease • Microstomia • Atrophy and induration of the skin • Contractures • Involvement of internal organs (lung, kidneys, bowel, heart) • Pulmonary symptoms occur as initial symptoms in less than 1% of patients (dyspnea, cough, chest pain).

▶ **Therapeutic options**
No curative therapy • Cytostatic and immunosuppressive agents can slow the progress of the disease • Cyclophosphamide is indicated for pulmonary involvement.

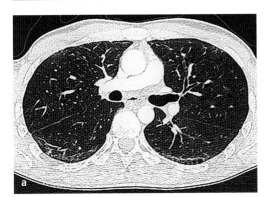

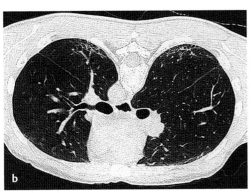

Fig. 6.6 Scleroderma in a 34-year-old man. The CT scans show relatively discrete and fine subpleural interstitial shadowing in the posterobasal segments of the lower lobes. The prone scans show these to be actual changes. This case does not exhibit any apparent esophageal dilatation.

Fig. 6.7 CT scans in a 55-year-old man. There is progressive systemic sclerosis. Severe interstitial fibrosis with primarily reticular and streaky changes accompanied by partially cystic and honeycombed parenchymal remodeling.

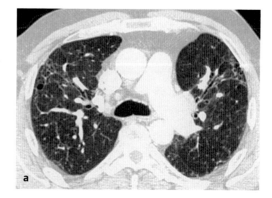

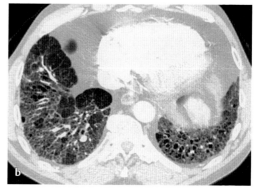

▶ **Course and prognosis**
Variable, usually poor (5-year survival rate is 70%) • Pulmonary involvement is usually the limiting factor.

▶ **What does the clinician want to know?**
Detection and evaluation of pulmonary changes.

Differential Diagnosis

Other collagen vascular diseases	– Not clearly distinguishable on the basis of pulmonary changes – Rheumatoid arthritis: no esophageal dilatation, presence of rheumatoid nodules and occasionally cavitation – Systemic lupus erythematosus: pleural and/or pericardial effusion, parenchymal consolidations
Idiopathic pulmonary fibrosis	– Coarser reticular shadowing and honeycombing – No esophageal dilatation
Nonspecific interstitial pneumonitis	– Morphologically indistinguishable – No esophageal dilatation
Asbestosis	– Pleural plaques – Subpleural linear opacities and parenchymal bands – No bronchiolectasis

Tips and Pitfalls

Where the underlying disorder is known, interpretation of the pulmonary findings is straightforward.

Selected References

Arroglia AC, Podell DN, Matthay RA. Pulmonary manifestations of scleroderma. J Thorac Imaging 1992; 7: 30–45

Bhalla M et al. Chest CT in patiens with scleroderma: prevalence of asymptomatic esophageal dilatation and mediastinal lymphadenopathy. AJR Am J Roentgenol 1993; 161: 269–272

Ostojic P et al. Interstitial lung disease in systemic sclerosis. Lung 2007; 185: 211–220

Definition

Polymyositis is a systemic inflammatory disorder of skeletal muscle; in dermatomyositis the skin is also involved.

▶ **Epidemiology**
  Women are affected twice as often as men.
▶ **Etiology, pathophysiology, pathogenesis**
  Associated with antinuclear and anticytoplasmic antibodies • Pulmonary involvement is rare • The disorder can occur as paraneoplasia (5–15% of patients who develop the disease have a malignancy).

Imaging Signs

▶ **Modality of choice**
  CT.
▶ **CT findings**
  Pulmonary involvement is rare (5–10% of cases) • Nonspecific interstitial changes include ground-glass opacity (90% of these cases), finely reticular shadowing (90%), consolidations (50%), honeycombing (15%) • Predominantly basal and subpleural findings.
▶ **Pathognomonic findings**
  Nonspecific interstitial changes predominantly in the basal and subpleural regions.

Clinical Aspects

▶ **Typical presentation**
  Muscle weakness and pain especially in the upper extremity • Signs of inflammation • Findings in polymyositis with dermatomyositis also include facial exanthema and eczematous dermatitis • Pulmonary changes (dyspnea, infiltrates) can precede the skin and muscle changes.
▶ **Therapeutic options**
  Immunosuppression.
▶ **Course and prognosis**
  Complete resolution occurs in about half of the cases • Prognosis depends on the organs involved (heart, lung).

Differential Diagnosis

Other collagen vascular diseases	– Clinical findings are crucial to the diagnosis
	– Morphologic findings on the radiograph are usually ambiguous
Sarcoidosis	– Usually associated with lymphadenopathy
	– Different clinical picture

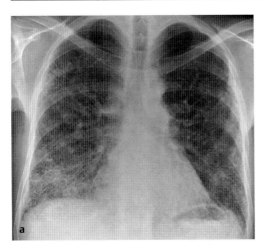

Fig. 6.8 Jo-1 syndrome, a variant of polymyositis with dermatomyositis, in a 46-year-old man.

a The plain chest radiograph shows severe reticulonodular and honeycomb shadowing with an increasing apicobasal gradient.

b These changes appear primarily as honeycomb structures on CT.

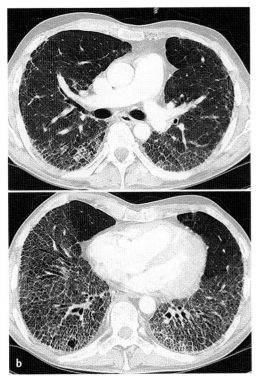

Selected References

Arakawa H et al. Nonspecific interstitial pneumonia associated with polymyositis and dermatomyositis: serial high-resolution CT findings and functional correlation. Chest 2003; 123: 1096–1103

Mino M et al. Pulmonary involvement in polymyositis and dermatomyositis: sequential evaluation with CT. AJR Am J Roentgenol 1997; 169: 83–87

Seiberlich B et al. Das Jo-1-Syndrom und seine klinischen Manifestationen. Med Klin 2005; 100: 137–142

Definition

Necrotizing granulomatous vasculitis.

▶ **Epidemiology**
Incidence is 7 : 10 000 per year • Primarily affects Caucasians • Most often occurs at age 30–50 years • No sex predilection.

▶ **Etiology, pathophysiology, pathogenesis**
Disorder of uncertain etiology involving multiple organ systems • Necrotizing vasculitis with granulomatous changes • Manifests itself in the lung and airways in about 90% of cases, kidneys in about 80%, joints in about 60%, skin in about 45%, and nerves in about 20%.

Imaging Signs

▶ **Modality of choice**
Radiographs, CT.

▶ **Radiographic findings**
Bilateral, well-demarcated, focal pulmonary lesions varying in number (1 to > 10) and size (2 cm to > 4 cm) with and without liquefaction (usually thick-walled cysts) • Consolidating shadows may be present • Subglottic stenosis.

▶ **CT findings**
In addition to radiographic findings, findings include halo sign in perifocal hemorrhage • Wedge-shaped consolidations due to infarction • Tracheobronchial changes include wall thickening, stenosis in 15–25% of cases • Pleural or pericardial effusion in about 20% • Signs of activity include liquefaction and necrosis, large focal lesions > 3 cm (foci < 15 mm are usually residual findings after treatment), consolidations, ground-glass opacities.

▶ **Pathognomonic findings**
Cavitary pulmonary focal lesions in combination with tracheal stenosis.

Clinical Aspects

▶ **Typical presentation**
  – Wegener triad of sinus, pulmonary, and renal manifestation.
  – *Initial stage (limited to the upper respiratory tract):* Sinusitis • Rhinitis • Otitis.
  – *Generalized stage:* Cough, dyspnea, hemoptysis • Hematuria, proteinuria • General symptoms include decreased exercise tolerance, symptoms of hepatitis B • Joint pain, neurologic symptoms, skin changes.
  – Up to 90% of patients are c-ANCA positive (although not an invariable finding).

▶ **Confirmation of the diagnosis**
Biopsy (lung, paranasal sinuses).

▶ **Therapeutic options**
Immunosuppressives (steroids, cyclophosphamide).

Fig. 6.9 Wegener granulomatosis in a 30-year-old woman. The plain chest radiograph and CT show several round focal lesions of varying size, some with liquefaction. No reaction in adjacent tissue.

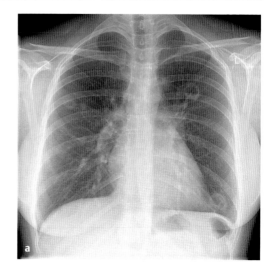

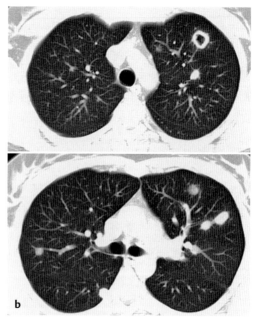

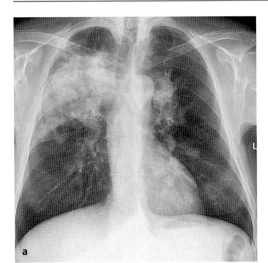

Fig. 6.10 Wegener granulomatosis in a 52-year-old man. Tumor-like consolidation in the right upper lobe. Similar, less extensive infiltrates are also visualized on the left.

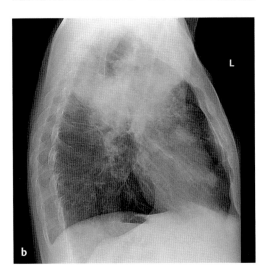

▶ **Course and prognosis**

Typically exhibits a two-phase course (initial stage and generalized stage) ● Symptoms usually remit rapidly (within a month) under treatment ● Rate of recurrence is 50% ● Most common cause of death is kidney failure.

▶ **What does the clinician want to know?**

Extent of organ manifestation ● Disease activity ● Course under therapy.

Differential Diagnosis

Mycosis, tuberculosis	– Can exhibit identical radiographic morphology – Differential diagnosis requires clinical and microbiologic data
Septic embolisms	– Rapid development – Clinical and microbiologic findings (blood culture)
Bronchial carcinoma (squamous cell carcinoma)	– Differential diagnosis requires clinical and histologic data
Metastases (squamous cell carcinoma, sarcoma)	– Differential diagnosis requires clinical and histologic data
Rheumatoid nodules	– Joint disease (history)

Tips and Pitfalls

Findings can be misinterpreted as pneumonic infiltrate, tumor, or metastases ● Tracheobronchial manifestations (subglottic stenosis) are often missed.

Selected References

Frazier AA et al. Pulmonary angiitis and granulomatosis: radiographic-pathologic correlation. Radiographics 1998; 18: 687–710

Lohrmann C et al. Pulmonary manifestations of Wegener granulomatosis: CT findings in 57 patients and a review of the literature. Eur J Radiol 2005; 53: 471–477

Definition

Hypersensitivity reaction to *Aspergillus* spores with mucoid impaction.

▶ **Epidemiology**
Most common bronchopulmonary mycosis in humans ● Affects younger adults (ages 20–40; women slightly more often than men) ● Atopic patients with bronchial asthma or in the setting of cystic fibrosis (occurs in 10% of cystic fibrosis patients, 1–2% of asthma patients).

▶ **Etiology, pathophysiology, pathogenesis**
Type I or III hypersensitivity reaction in the bronchial system and the adjacent lung tissue ● Leads to cystic-varicose bronchiectasis.

Imaging Signs

▶ **Modality of choice**
CT is preferable to plain radiography.

▶ **Radiographic and CT findings**
Linear shadow bands bifurcate to form V- or Y-shaped figures (bronchoceles, i.e., cystic mucus-filled bronchiectatic areas); there may be fluid shadows ● Mucus obstruction causes atelectasis ● Transient eosinophilic infiltrates ● Predilection for the proximal bronchial areas, and the upper and middle lung fields.

▶ **Pathognomonic findings**
Bifurcating linear shadow bands ● "Finger in glove" and "toothpaste" shadows.

Clinical Aspects

▶ **Typical presentation**
Chronic recurrent asthma ● Cough with viscous sputum ● Hemoptysis ● Eosinophilia ● Hyphae in the sputum ● Antigen reaction.

▶ **Therapeutic options**
Steroids.

▶ **Course and prognosis**
Variable ● Recurrent allergic bronchopulmonary aspergillosis leads to central bronchiectasis and fibrosis in the upper field.

▶ **What does the clinician want to know?**
Suspected diagnosis.

Differential Diagnosis

Cystic fibrosis and/or bronchiectasis	– No blood eosinophilia – Generalized changes and known underlying disorder in cystic fibrosis
Bronchial atresia	– Usually in the apical posterior left upper lobe – Increased transradiancy and diminished vascularity – No history of allergy or cystic fibrosis

Fig. 7.1 Allergic bronchopulmonary aspergillosis in a 10-year-old girl with cystic fibrosis. The plain chest radiograph shows pronounced bronchial walls in the perihilar region and in the lower lung fields with faint bronchiectasis in the right middle lung field. Findings in the left upper lung field include an area of opacity that appears to "branch" peripherally. A similar, round pleural opacity is also seen nearby. These findings correspond to confluent areas of tubular impaction in allergic bronchopulmonary aspergillosis.

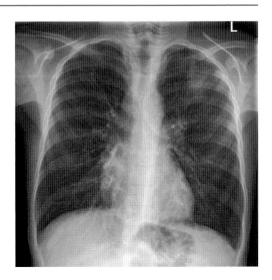

| *Bronchocentric granulomatosis* | – Solitary or multiple sublobular consolidations in close proximity to the airways, usually unilaterally in the upper fields |
| | – Where asthma is present, findings are indistinguishable from allergic bronchopulmonary aspergillosis |

Tips and Pitfalls

Findings are nonspecific.

Selected References

Franquet T et al. Spectrum of pulmonary aspergillosis: histologic, clinical, and radiologic findings. Radiographics 2001; 21: 825–837

Johkoh T et al. Eosinophilic lung diseases: diagnostic accuracy of thin section CT in 111 patients. Radiology 2000; 216: 773–780

Ward S et al. Accuracy of CT in the diagnosis of allergic bronchopulmonary aspergillosis in asthmatic patients. AJR Am J Roentgenol 1999; 173: 937–942

Definition

Immune reaction of the alveoli and bronchioles to inhalation of toxic substances •
Synonym: Organic dust toxic syndrome.

▶ **Epidemiology**
Typical constellations are named after the specific type of exposure • Farmer's
lung (thermophilic actinomycetes) • Pigeon breeder's lung (proteins) • Ventilator
pneumonitis or Monday morning fever (heat tolerant bacteria), etc.

▶ **Etiology, pathophysiology, pathogenesis**
Allergic granulomatous reaction (bronchiolitis and alveolitis) • Inhalation of ani-
mal proteins, pathogenic microorganisms, spores, mineral oils, chemical organic
substances (measuring 1–5 μm) • Prerequisite is an individual predisposition • In
the acute stage there is bronchiolitis with proliferation of alveolar cells • Subacute
stage involves development of interstitial granulomas • The chronic stage includes development of interstitial fibrosis, honeycomb lung, and cysts.

Imaging Signs

▶ **Modality of choice**
CT.

▶ **Radiographic findings**
Findings are usually normal in the acute and subacute stages • Rarely, there will
be discrete ground-glass opacities or nodular and reticulonodular changes • The
chronic stage includes fibrosis predominantly in the middle field that spares the
costophrenic angle.

▶ **CT findings**
 – *Acute and subacute stages:* Disseminated, ill-defined centrilobular nodules that
   can resemble ground-glass lesions • Diffuse or nodular ground-glass opacity •
   Predominantly in the middle and lower lung fields.
 – *Chronic stage:* Honeycomb fibrosis, cystic changes, traction bronchiectasis, and
   volume loss • No pleural or subpleural involvement • No lymphadenopathy.

▶ **Pathognomonic findings**
In the subacute phase these include diffuse and nodular ground-glass opacities,
ill-defined centrilobular nodules (acinar nodules), predominantly in the middle
and lower lung fields • Later findings include fibrotic changes, acinar nodules,
and ground-glass opacities.

Clinical Aspects

▶ **Typical presentation**
The acute stage (4–8 hours after exposure) is characterized by flulike symptoms,
nonproductive cough with dyspnea, resolving within 1–2 weeks • The subacute
chronic stage manifests as recurrent, episodic, and progressive shortness of
breath (a sign of restrictive and obstructive pulmonary dysfunction).

Fig. 7.2 Acute stage of extrinsic allergic alveolitis in a 45-year-old woman.
a The plain chest radiograph shows no abnormal findings.
b CT shows ground-glass opacification uniformly involving all lung segments.

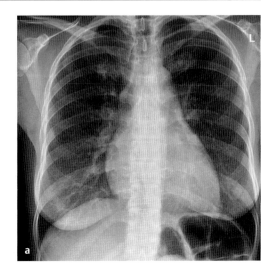

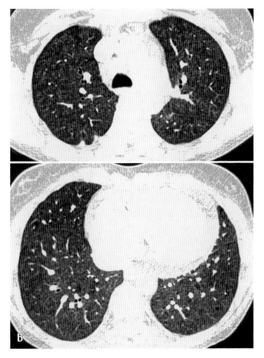

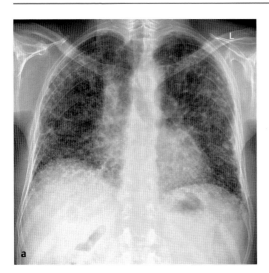

Fig. 7.3 Severe fibrosis of the lung within the framework of an extrinsic allergic alveolitis in a 60-year-old man (birdkeeper). Fibrosis with cystic parenchym alterations. Traction bronchiectasy, widening of the central tracheobronchial system and decreased lung volume, encapsulated pneumothorax on the right.

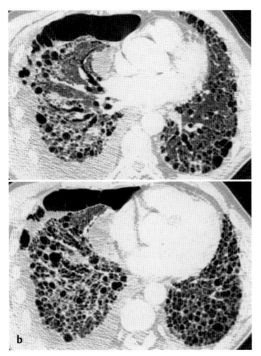

▶ **Diagnostic criteria**

History (antigen exposure and time-dependent symptoms), specifically immunoglobulin G (IgG) antibodies, radiographic findings, decreased pO_2 • Diagnosis is confirmed by bronchoalveolar lavage and by bronchial provocation testing where indicated.

▶ **Therapeutic options**

Prophylaxis against exposure • Steroids.

▶ **Course and prognosis**

Variable • Prognosis is good with prompt diagnosis and prophylaxis against exposure.

▶ **What does the clinician want to know?**

Extent of organ manifestation • Disease activity • Course under therapy.

Differential Diagnosis

Toxic alveolitis	– Normal radiographic findings – No pulmonary dysfunction or impaired diffusion – No antibodies
Bronchopulmonary infection	– History – Course under antibiotics – Bronchoalveolar lavage
Nonspecific interstitial pneumonitis	– Ground-glass opacities – Peribronchovascular distribution – No honeycombing – Histologic examination recommended to exclude extrinsic allergic alveolitis
Respiratory bronchiolitis with interstitial lung disease	– Smoker – Centrilobular emphysema – Primarily in the upper lobes
Silicosis	– History of occupational exposure
Sarcoidosis	– Peribronchovascular distribution – Lymphadenopathy
Scleroderma	– Predominantly basal fibrosis – Esophageal dilatation

Tips and Pitfalls

The acute stage is often misdiagnosed as a flulike infection • The chronic stage is indistinguishable from other chronic inflammatory pulmonary disorders.

Selected References

Lynch DA et al. Can CT distinguish hypersensitivity pneumonitis from idiopathic pulmonary fibrosis? AJR Am J Roentgenol 1995; 165: 807–811

Matar LD, McAdams HP, Sporn TA. Hypersensitivity pneumonitis. AJR Am J Roentgenol 2000; 174: 1061–1066

Sennekamp J, Müller-Wening D. [Exogen-allergische Alveolitis.] Pneumologe 2006; 3: 461–470 [In German]

Definition

A group of etiologically and clinically heterogeneous disorders with tissue eosinophilia and usually but not invariably blood eosinophilia—Loeffler infiltrate • Acute eosinophilic pneumonia • Chronic eosinophilic pneumonia • Idiopathic hypereosinophilic syndrome.

▶ **Epidemiology**
Chronic eosinophilic pneumonia is often associated with atopic disorders (especially asthma) • Women are affected twice as often as men • Peak occurrence at age 30–40 years • Hypereosinophilia syndrome is more common in men than women by a ratio of 7 : 1.

▶ **Etiology, pathophysiology, pathogenesis**
Etiology is either unclear or reactive secondary to drugs, parasites (ascarids, amebas), fungi, etc. • Morphologic findings include edema, and alveolar and interstitial eosinophilic infiltrates.

Imaging Signs

▶ **Modality of choice**
CT is usually preferable to plain radiography.

▶ **Radiographic and CT findings**
 – *Loeffler syndrome:* Ill-defined transient or migrating nonsegmental infiltrates • CT shows ground-glass or denser foci with halos.
 – *Acute eosinophilic pneumonia:* Bilateral reticular and nodular nonsegmental opacities • CT shows ground-glass opacities.
 – *Chronic eosinophilic pneumonia:* Homogeneous peripheral subpleural shadows ("negative image" of the edema) persisting for months, bilateral in 50% of cases, nonsegmental, predilection for the upper lobe, air bronchogram may be present • Resolves leaving bandlike densities parallel to the pleura • CT allows better evaluation of the characteristic topology.
 – *Idiopathic hypereosinophilic syndrome:* Loeffler-like picture but persistent, due at least partially to cardiac involvement • Pleural effusion occurs in 50% of cases.

▶ **Pathognomonic findings**
 – *Acute eosinophilic pneumonia:* Edemalike infiltrates.
 – *Chronic eosinophilic pneumonia:* Peripheral subpleural shadows ("negative image" of the edema) which resolve leaving bandlike densities parallel to the pleura.
 – *Loeffler syndrome:* Transient infiltrates with halo.
 – *Idiopathic hypereosinophilic syndrome:* Nodular infiltrates with halo.

Clinical Aspects

▶ **Typical presentation**
 – *Loeffler syndrome:* Minimally symptomatic.
 – *Acute eosinophilic pneumonia:* Fever • Dyspnea • Myalgia • Malaise • Blood eosinophilia is not invariably present.

Fig. 7.4 Eosinophilic pneumonia in a 54-year-old man.

a The plain chest radiograph shows partially fine nodular and partially streaky reticular shadowing bilaterally and primarily in the basal region.

b Similar changes seen on CT, except that the nodular opacities appear as focal ground-glass opacities.

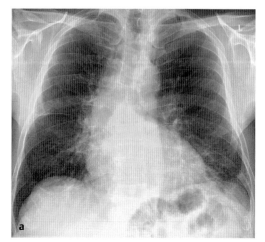

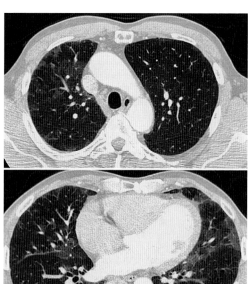

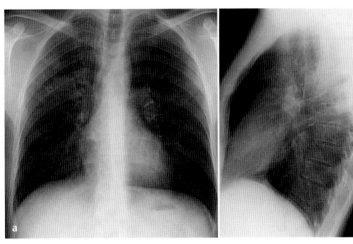

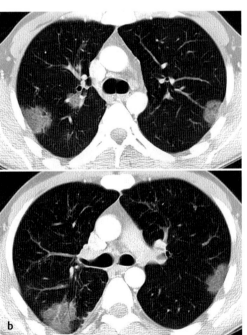

Fig. 7.5 Eosinophilic pneumonia in a 34-year-old man. The plain chest radiographs and CT show patchy, minimally dense infiltrates with pleural involvement in both upper lobes.

– *Chronic eosinophilic pneumonia:* Fever • Dyspnea • Cough • Asthma is present in 50% of cases.
– *Idiopathic hypereosinophilic syndrome:* Long history • Severe eosinophilia • Involves multiple organ systems (heart more than lung).

▶ **Therapeutic options**
Simple pulmonary eosinophilia usually resolves spontaneously • Corticosteroids are indicated in the other idiopathic eosinophilic disorders.

▶ **Course and prognosis**
Simple pulmonary eosinophilia has a good prognosis even without treatment • Acute and chronic eosinophilic pneumonia and hypereosinophilic syndrome have a good prognosis with steroid therapy • Recurrence is rare in acute eosinophilic pneumonia but common in chronic eosinophilic pneumonia.

▶ **What does the clinician want to know?**
Diagnosis • Course.

Differential Diagnosis

Churg–Strauss syndrome	– Morphologically indistinguishable
	– Migrating multifocal consolidations and ground-glass opacities, especially peripherally
	– Pulmonary nodules
	– Hemorrhages
	– Thickening of the bronchial wall or bronchiectasis
	– Septal thickening
	– Pleural effusions
Idiopathic hypereosinophilic	– Transient ground-glass opacities
	– Consolidations
	– Bilateral, primarily peripheral nodules up to 1 cm in size
	– With cardiac involvement there may also be signs of pulmonary edema
Other pulmonary disorders and reactions involving eosinophilia	– Allergic bronchopulmonary aspergillosis
	– Bronchocentric granulomatosis
	– Parasites (ascarids, filariae, amebas): history and diagnosis of exclusion
	– Drug reaction: history and diagnosis of exclusion

Tips and Pitfalls

Can be misinterpreted as pneumonia.

Selected References

Jeong YJ et al. Eosinophilic lung diseases: a clinical, radiologic, and pathologic overview. Radiographics 2007; 27: 617–639

Johkoh T et al. Eosinophilic lung diseases: diagnostic accuracy of thin-section CT in 111 patients. Radiology 2000; 216: 773–780

Definition

Diffuse pulmonary and alveolar hemorrhages from various causes.

▶ **Epidemiology**

The most common cause is Goodpasture syndrome (affects young adults, more common in men than women by a ratio of 9 : 1) ● Less common causes include collagen vascular diseases (more common in women than men), idiopathic disease (pulmonary hemosiderosis), hemorrhagic diathesis, and diffuse coagulation disorder.

▶ **Etiology, pathophysiology, pathogenesis**

Bleeding into the alveoli due to immune-mediated capillary damage (antibodies to glomerular and alveolar basement membranes in Goodpasture syndrome) or due to nonimmune-mediated capillary damage ● Leads successively to recurrent hemorrhage, hemosiderin deposits, and fibrosis.

Imaging Signs

▶ **Modality of choice**

CT is preferable to plain radiography.

▶ **Radiographic findings**

Nodular, confluent to patchy, edemalike shadows ● Predominantly basal and central ● In the acute stage there is alveolar shadowing ● In the subacute stage there is an interstitial reticulonodular pattern ● Resolves within 1–2 weeks ● Chronic stage (recurrent hemorrhages) leads to fibrosis.

▶ **CT findings**

Findings in the acute stage include ill-defined acinar nodules, circumscribed ground-glass opacities, or diffuse bilateral consolidation that spares the pulmonary periphery ● The subacute stage includes micronodules and septal thickening ● In the chronic stage there are signs of fibrosis.

▶ **Pathognomonic findings on CT**

Acute nodular or interstitial shadowing that rapidly resolves spontaneously.

Clinical Aspects

▶ **Typical presentation**

Hemoptysis (in 80% of cases but not invariably), dyspnea, cough, and iron-deficiency anemia ● Goodpasture syndrome also includes hematuria, renal insufficiency, hypertension ● Bronchoalveolar lavage shows hemosiderin-laden macrophages.

▶ **Therapeutic options**

Treatment of the underlying disorder ● Immunosuppressives ● Glucocorticoids ● Plasmapheresis.

▶ **Course and prognosis**

Variable ● Depend on the underlying disorder.

▶ **What does the clinician want to know?**

Diagnosis and differential diagnosis ● Stage ● Follow-up.

Fig. 7.6   Goodpasture syndrome in a 35-year-old man. The CT scans show bilateral, homogeneously dense, ground-glass opacification that has spared only the sub-pleural parenchyma.

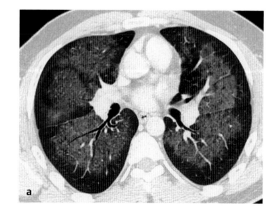

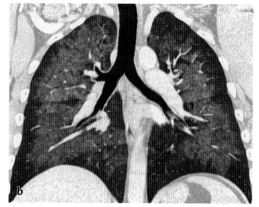

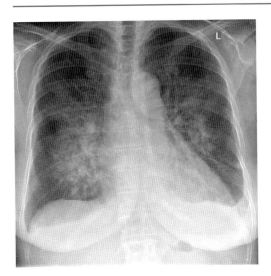

Fig. 7.7 Acute pulmonary hemorrhage in a 70-year-old woman with dyspnea and hemoptysis. Moderately dense, homogeneous, bilateral perihilar and basal shadows resembling a butterfly edema.

Differential Diagnosis

Pulmonary hemorrhage	– Goodpasture syndrome: antibodies to basement membrane
	– Wegener granulomatosis: ANCA-positive involvement of the paranasal sinuses
	– Churg–Strauss syndrome: asthma, blood eosinophilia
	– Systemic lupus erythematosus: ANCA-positive
	– Polyangiitis: pulmonary and renal syndrome, fever, myalgia, joint pain, 80% of patients are ANCA-positive
	– Idiopathic hemosiderosis: occurs in children, no renal involvement, no antibodies
Pulmonary edema (cardiac, not cardiac)	– Hemoptysis rare
	– Associated pleural effusion
Interstitial pneumonia	– Fever, inflammation parameters
	– No hemoptysis
	– No renal involvement

Tips and Pitfalls

Can be misinterpreted as pulmonary edema or atypical pneumonia.

Selected References

Cheah FK, Sheppard MN, Hansell DM. Computed tomography of diffuse pulmonary haemorrhage with pathological correlation. Clin Radiol 1993; 48: 89–93

Marten K et al. Pattern-based differential diagnosis in pulmonary vasculitis using volumetric CT. AJR Am J Roentgenol 2005; 184: 720–733

Definition

▶ **Epidemiology**
Recurrent episodes of pulmonary bleeding without associated glomerulonephritis or serologic changes.

▶ **Etiology, pathophysiology, pathogenesis**
The cause is not fully understood; a genetic component has been postulated • The acute form is rare, affecting men twice as often as women • The chronic form usually affects children under 10 years • Bleeding from the alveolar capillaries into the pulmonary parenchyma leads to accumulation of hemoglobin and subsequently hemosiderin deposits in this area; hemosiderin-laden macrophages induce an inflammatory reaction.

Imaging Signs

▶ **Modality of choice**
Radiographs, CT.

▶ **Radiographic and CT findings**
Depending on severity, findings in the acute phase (hemorrhage stage) range from nodular alveolar shadowing and ground-glass opacification to confluent shadowing with or without an air bronchogram • The perihilar and basal regions are primarily affected, whereas the apex of the lung is usually spared • Lesions resolve within a few days.
Chronic recurrent hemorrhages lead to irreversible but discrete interstitial fibrosis without disorganization of pulmonary architecture, visualized on CT • These findings may be masked by more recent hemorrhage.

▶ **Pathognomonic findings**
Acute, spontaneous occurrence of an edemalike picture with hemoptysis.

Clinical Aspects

▶ **Typical presentation**
Triad of hemoptysis, pulmonary infiltrates, and anemia • Severe hemorrhaging is associated with dyspnea, cough, tachypnea, fever • Bronchoalveolar lavage demonstrates siderophages.

▶ **Therapeutic options**
Steroids • Immunosuppression • Severe hemorrhage with airway obstruction may require endoscopic intervention to clear clot material or extracorporeal membrane oxygenation (ECMO).

▶ **Course and prognosis**
Left untreated, the disorder leads to pulmonary fibrosis with restrictive pulmonary dysfunction • Massive bleeding can be fatal • Prompt diagnosis and aggressive immunosuppression improve the prognosis • Mean survival time is 5–15 years.

▶ **What does the clinician want to know?**
Extent of findings.

Immune Disorders and Disorders of Uncertain Etiology

Fig. 7.8 Pulmonary interstitial process accompanied by recurrent pulmonary hemorrhages with dyspnea and hemoptysis. The plain chest radiograph shows discrete reticulonodular shadowing primarily in the perihilar and basal regions with signs of right heart strain.

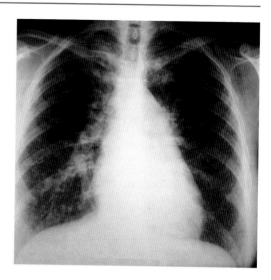

Differential Diagnosis

Goodpasture syndrome	– Glomerulonephritis – Findings include circulating antibodies to basement membranes
Secondary pulmonary hemorrhages in the setting of autoimmune and collagen vascular disorders	– Wegener granulomatosis: renal involvement, rhinitis, sinusitis, pulmonary nodules, and occasionally cavitations – Systemic lupus erythematosus: progressive respiratory failure, serum antinuclear antibodies, immune complexes in the lung biopsy
Bleeding secondary to trauma or biopsy	– History

Tips and Pitfalls

Can be misinterpreted as edema • Radiographic morphology provides no etiologic information and is indistinguishable from secondary pulmonary hemorrhage.

Selected References

Nuesslein TG, Teig N, Rieger CHL. Pulmonary haemosiderosis in children and infants. Paediatr Respir Rev 2006; 7: 45–48

Primack SL, Miller RR, Müller NL. Diffuse pulmonary hemorrhage: Clinical, pathologic and imaging features. AJR Am J Roentgenol 1995; 164: 295–300

Definition

Systemic granulomatosis of unknown etiology.

▶ **Epidemiology**

Common, often asymptomatic pulmonary disorder ● Can involve multiple organ systems ● Prognosis depends on pulmonary involvement.

▶ **Etiology, pathophysiology, pathogenesis**

Systemic disorder of uncertain etiology ● Lungs are involved in 90% of cases ● Forms noncaseating granulomas ● Occurs between the ages of 20 and 40 years ● More common in women than in men.

Imaging Signs

▶ **Modality of choice**

CT is preferable to plain radiography.

▶ **Radiographic findings**

Bilateral hilar and mediastinal (paratracheal) lymphomas (in 80% of cases) ● *Pulmonary changes* (in 20%): Reticulonodular focal lesions, infiltrates with air bronchogram, fibrotic changes ● Radiographic findings are normal in 10% of cases.

▶ **CT findings**

Nodular focal lesions (1–5 mm) with a centrilobular, perivascular, and perilymphatic pattern of distribution ● Focal lesions occurring in clusters or along the bronchovascular bundles are a relatively characteristic finding ● Predilection for the posterior upper lobe and apical lower lobe ● Less characteristic findings include consolidations with an air bronchogram, fibrosis with cyst formation, and traction bronchiectasis.

▶ **Pathognomonic findings**

Symmetric bilateral hilar and mediastinal (paratracheal) lymphadenopathy ● Granulomatous pulmonary changes ● In the late stage, fibrosis predominantly in the upper lobe.

Clinical Aspects

▶ **Typical presentation**

Asymptomatic incidental finding or reduced exercise tolerance, weight loss, fever, cough ● Erythema nodosum ● Uveitis ● Arthritis.

▶ **Therapeutic options**

Steroids ● Mild cases do not require treatment.

▶ **Course and prognosis**

In the majority of cases the prognosis is good with complete remission within 2 years ● Irreversible fibrosis develops in about 20%.

▶ **What does the clinician want to know?**

Staging (stage 0 = no abnormal findings; stage 1 = bilateral hilar lymphadenopathy; stage 2 = bilateral hilar lymphadenopathy, lung changes; stage 3 = lung changes only; stage 4 = irreversible fibrosis).

Fig. 7.9 Sarcoidosis with pulmonary involvement (stage II–III) in a 36-year-old man with pain in the left chest without dyspnea or fever.

a The plain chest radiograph shows bilateral hilar lymphadenopathy and finely nodular shadowing primarily in the upper and middle lung fields.

b,c CT confirms the above findings.

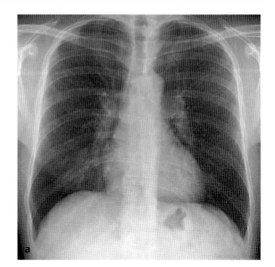

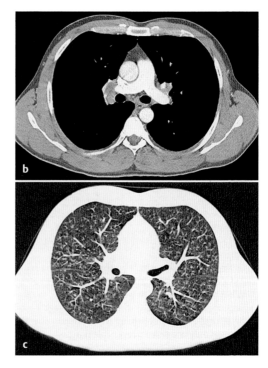

Immune Disorders and Disorders of Uncertain Etiology

Differential Diagnosis

Differential diagnosis depends on the form of manifestation of sarcoidosis • Lymphadenopathy versus pulmonary changes.

Idiopathic pulmonary fibrosis	– No lymphadenopathy
Langerhans cell histiocytosis	– Absent or minimal lymphadenopathy – Cysts
Pneumoconiosis	– History of exposure
Tuberculosis	– Asymmetric lymphadenopathy – Infiltrative changes – Pleural effusion – Miliary tuberculosis without lymphadenopathy
Mycoses	– Asymmetric lymphadenopathy – Opportunistic infection – Risk group
Lymphoma or lymph node metastases	– Asymmetric lymphadenopathy – Extrathoracic involvement – History of known malignancy

Tips and Pitfalls

Severe and advanced findings (fibrosis) are often not recognized as sarcoidosis when an underlying disorder has escaped detection to date.

Selected References

Hennebicque AS et al. CT findings in severe thoracic sarcoidosis. Eur Radiol 2005; 15: 23–30

Miller BH et al. Thoracic sarcoidosis: radiologic-pathologic correlation. Radiographics 1995; 15: 421–437

Traill ZC, Maskell GF, Gleeson FV. High-resolution CT findings of pulmonary sarcoidosis. AJR Am J Roentgenol 1997; 168: 1557–1560

Definition

Diffuse pulmonary disorder characterized by excessive deposition of proteinaceous lipid-rich surfactant material.

▶ **Epidemiology**

Very rare ● Peak occurrence is between the ages of 20 and 40 years ● Men are affected twice as often as women.

▶ **Etiology, pathophysiology, pathogenesis**

Primary forms are of unknown etiology; genetic mutation has been postulated ● Secondary forms occur in immune defects, hematologic disorders, exposure to silicate dust ● Deranged surfactant metabolism with alveolar accumulation of phospholipid or proteinaceous surfactant components leads to obstruction of the gas-exchanging surface.

Imaging Signs

▶ **Modality of choice**

CT.

▶ **Radiographic findings**

Bilateral, approximately symmetric alveolar shadow, more pronounced in the center ("bat wing" sign) ● There may be a faint air bronchogram.

▶ **CT findings**

Findings include areas of normal parenchyma alternating with maplike areas in which polygonal fields of ground-glass opacification and septal thickening produce a "crazy paving" pattern ● No pleural effusion or lymphadenopathy is seen (except in superinfection).

▶ **Pathognomonic findings on CT**

"Crazy paving" pattern is typical but not pathognomonic ● Lavage findings are diagnostic.

Clinical Aspects

▶ **Typical presentation**

Two-thirds of cases involve progressive dyspnea, cough (reduced DLCO), and weight loss ● One-third are asymptomatic ● Often severe radiographic findings contrast with milder clinical symptoms.

▶ **Confirmation of the diagnosis**

Bronchoalveolar lavage or biopsy.

▶ **Therapeutic options**

Primary disease is treated by therapeutic bronchoalveolar lavage or lung transplantation ● Secondary disease is treated by therapeutic bronchoalveolar lavage, management of the underlying disorder, and prophylaxis against exposure.

▶ **Course and prognosis**

Prognosis is favorable ● 5-year survival is 80%.

▶ **What does the clinician want to know?**

Diagnosis and differential diagnosis ● Secondary complications ● Course.

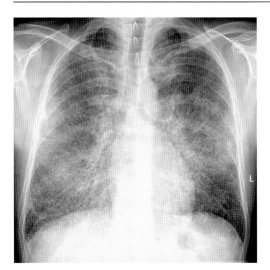

Fig. 7.10 Alveolar proteinosis in a 39-year-old man. The plain chest radiograph shows significant, primarily perihilar interstitial shadowing with opacification and masking of vascular structures.

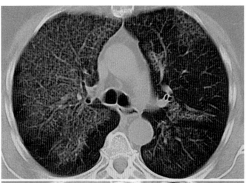

Fig. 7.11 Alveolar proteinosis in a 58-year-old woman with fever and cough with sputum persisting over several months. CT shows nearly symmetric areas of ground-glass opacification exhibiting a faint "crazy paving" pattern of polygonal fields and sparing the periphery.

Immune Disorders and Disorders of Uncertain Etiology

Differential Diagnosis

Pulmonary edema	– Pleural effusion
	– Responds to medication
Pulmonary hemorrhage	– Morphologically not clearly distinguishable
	– Anemia
	– Hemoptysis
Pneumonia	– Segmental or lobar distribution
	– Fever
	– Laboratory diagnostic tests
	– Isolated pathogen
	– *Pneumocystis jirovecii* pneumonia can show "crazy paving" pattern
Bronchioalveolar carcinoma	– Morphologically not clearly distinguishable

Tips and Pitfalls

Exclude bronchioalveolar carcinoma.

Selected References

Albafouille V, Sayegh N, De Coudenhove S. CT scan patterns of pulmonary alveolar proteinosis in children. Pediatr Radiol 1999; 29: 147–152

Bewig B et al. GM-CSF and GM-CSF bc receptor in adult patients with pulmonary alveolar proteinosis. Eur Respir J 2000; 15: 350–357

Prakash UB et al. Pulmonary alveolar phospholipoproteinosis: experience with 34 cases and a review. Mayo Clin Proc 1987; 62: 499–518

Definition

Cystic destruction of pulmonary parenchyma due to proliferation of atypical muscle cells.

▶ **Epidemiology**
Very rare • Occurs exclusively in women of childbearing age • Identical pulmonary pathology as in tuberous sclerosis (1% of cases).

▶ **Etiology, pathophysiology, pathogenesis**
Etiology is unknown • Sex and age distribution suggests a hormonal cause (estrogens) • Proliferation of smooth muscle cells around lymph and blood vessels and bronchi with cystic destruction of pulmonary parenchyma.

Imaging Signs

▶ **Modality of choice**
CT.

▶ **Radiographic findings**
Findings in the early stages are often normal; may include discrete thin-walled cysts • Later, the summation of cyst walls creates an irregular reticular pattern • No volume loss • Usually slight, chylous pleural effusion.

▶ **CT**
Initial findings include thin-walled cysts of nearly uniform size and distribution in all lung fields • These are interspersed with normal lung tissue • Advanced stages exhibit cysts increasing in number and size (2 mm to > 10 mm) until they have largely replaced the parenchyma • Chylous pleural effusion occurs in 60% of cases • Mediastinal lymphadenopathy in 50%.

▶ **Pathognomonic findings**
Disseminated, uniformly distributed thin-walled cysts in otherwise normal pulmonary parenchyma with associated pleural effusion in a young woman.

Clinical Aspects

▶ **Typical presentation**
Nonspecific symptoms with dyspnea, which is why the disorder is often diagnosed only years later • Spontaneous pneumothorax • Chylous pleural effusion • Hemoptysis due to pulmonary hemorrhage.

▶ **Therapeutic options**
Adnexectomy and progesterone substitution • Pleurodesis • Lung transplant.

▶ **Course and prognosis**
Progressive respiratory insufficiency • 5-year survival rate is about 50%.

▶ **What does the clinician want to know?**
Diagnosis and/or differential diagnosis • HRCT findings are diagnostic in the presence of appropriate clinical findings.

Fig. 7.12 Lymphangio-leiomyomatosis in a 45-year-old woman, diagnosed during bullectomy for recurrent pneumothorax.

a The plain chest radiograph does not show any obvious abnormal findings.

b CT shows isolated small cystic changes uniformly distributed throughout both lungs in otherwise normal parenchyma. The cysts are thin-walled. No pleural effusion or lymphadenopathy.

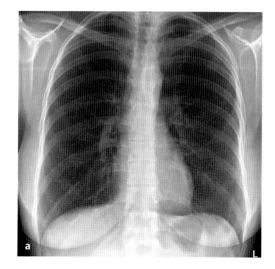

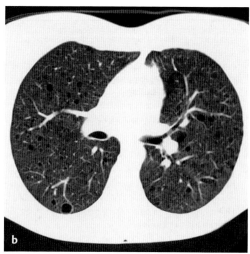

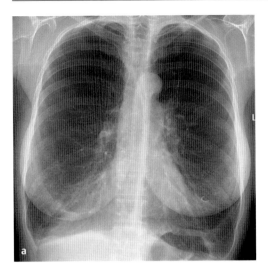

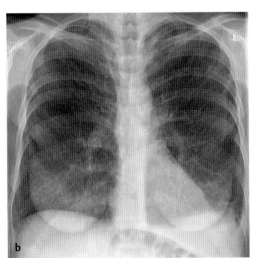

Fig. 7.13 Two cases of lymphangioleiomyomatosis with different radiographic morphology.
a 52-year-old woman. The radiograph predominantly shows an emphysema-like picture with significantly diminished vascularity and a low-lying flattened diaphragm.
b 29-year-old woman. Severe interstitial changes with a primarily reticular cystic pattern and uniform involvement of all lung segments. Associated left basal pleural effusion.

Differential Diagnosis

Langerhans cell histiocytosis	– The often irregular cystic changes are associated with centrilobular nodular changes – Lower lung fields are not involved – No pleural effusion – History of smoking
Panlobular emphysema	– No cyst wall – No pleural effusion – No sex predilection
Lymphocytic interstitial pneumonitis	– Combination of diffuse ground-glass opacities and predominantly subpleural thin-walled parenchymal cysts – Centrilobular nodular opacities and nodular consolidations

Tips and Pitfalls

Normal CT findings do not exclude lymphangioleiomyomatosis • Diagnosis is confirmed by biopsy.

Selected References

Sherrier RH, Chiles C, Roggli V. Pulmonary lymphangioleiomyomatosis: CT findings. AJR Am J Roentgenol 1989; 153: 937–940

Sullivan EJ. Lymphangioleiomyomatosis: a review. Chest 1998; 114: 1689–1703

Definition

Destruction of peripheral airways by "specific" granulomas.

▶ **Epidemiology**
Rare; incidence is about 10–15 : 10 000 per year • Accounts for about 4% of generalized lung disorders • Peak occurrence is at age 20–30 years • No sex predilection • In adults it is most often limited to one lung • In 30% of cases there is simultaneous skeletal and/or liver involvement.

▶ **Etiology, pathophysiology, pathogenesis**
Etiology is unknown • Linked to cigarette smoking • Destructive granulomatous inflammation of the pulmonary interstitium (primarily Langerhans cells) with formation of cysts and proliferative fibrosis in the terminal stage.

Imaging Signs

▶ **Modality of choice**
CT.

▶ **Radiographic findings**
Bilateral, disseminated, ill-defined reticulonodular opacities with cystic components • Shows a predilection for the upper and middle lung fields, sparing the lower fields • No pleural effusion.

▶ **CT findings**
Bilateral, partially nodular but primarily cystic changes in the upper and middle lung fields, sparing the costophrenic angle • Centrilobular and peribronchial nodular focal lesions measuring 1–10 mm; these may be irregular, solid, or show liquefaction • Bizarrely configured, lobulated, or septate cysts, 1–20 mm • Honeycomb lung from progressive parenchymal fibrosis • Ground-glass opacification is rarely present.

▶ **Pathognomonic findings**
Reticulonodular and cystic changes in the upper and middle lung fields in young smokers.

Clinical Aspects

▶ **Typical presentation**
Nonproductive cough • Dyspnea • Chest pain • Fever • Weight loss • Pneumothorax commonly occurs in subpleural cyst rupture (25% of cases) • 20% of cases are asymptomatic or minimally symptomatic.

▶ **Confirmation of the diagnosis**
Transbronchial or open biopsy.

▶ **Therapeutic options**
Tobacco abstinence • Spontaneous remission of pulmonary manifestations may occur • Steroids or chemotherapy are indicated for progressive disease • Terminal-stage disease requires a lung transplant.

Fig. 7.14 Langerhans cell histiocytosis in a 44-year-old woman. The pronounced, finely reticular shadowing over all lung fields on the plain chest radiograph (**a**) is visualized on CT as thin-walled cysts and reticular thickening of the interstitium without signs of nodular focal lesions (**b**).

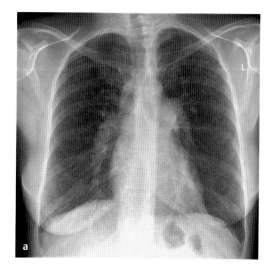

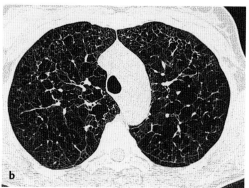

▶ **Course and prognosis**

Variable ● Depends on the pattern of involvement (one or more organs) ● Complete remission, nonprogressive disease, and respiratory insufficiency are possible ● Mortality is less than 5%.

▶ **What does the clinician want to know?**

Diagnosis and/or differential diagnosis ● Activity and course of the disease.

Differential Diagnosis

Lymphangioleiomyomatosis	– No nodular opacities – Uniformly round cysts – Involvement of all segments – Pleural effusion – Exclusively affects young women
Sarcoidosis	– No cystic changes – Mediastinal and/or hilar lymphadenopathy – Langerhans cell histiocytosis and sarcoidosis can present identical pictures in the terminal stage
Bullous emphysema	– Langerhans cell histiocytosis and bullous emphysema can present identical pictures in the terminal stage
Hypersensitivity pneumonia	– Nodules and distribution pattern are identical to Langerhans cell histiocytosis – Cystic lesions, but rarely and few

Tips and Pitfalls

In its terminal stages, the disease is radiographically indistinguishable from sarcoidosis or severe bullous emphysema.

Selected References

Brauner MW et al. Pulmonary Langerhans cell histiocytosis: evolution of lesions on CT scans. Radiology 1997; 204: 497–502

Moore AD et al. Pulmonary histiocytosis X: comparison of radiographic and CT findings. Radiology 1989; 172: 249–254

Definition
....

Primary neoplasms of the lung and bronchial system.

▶ **Epidemiology**

Most common cause of death from cancer • More common in men than women • Age 40–70 • A fundamental distinction is made between small cell lung cancer (SCLC, 15–20% of cases) and nonsmall cell lung cancer (NSCLC, 80–85%) • Adenocarcinoma is the most common type of nonsmall cell lung cancer (40%, acinar, papillary, bronchioalveolar, solid, mucus-forming), followed by squamous cell carcinoma (30%), and large cell carcinoma (15%).

▶ **Etiology, pathophysiology, pathogenesis**

Main risk factor is cigarette smoking; other factors include asbestos exposure.

Imaging Signs
....

▶ **Modality of choice**

CT (including the adrenal region), PET (PET/CT) • Chest radiographs are not used in staging.

▶ **Radiographic findings**

Pulmonary focal lesion of variable size (1–10 cm) with ill-defined margins and spicules • Larger focal lesions are often lobulated • Lesions occur more often in the upper lobe than lower lobe • Adenocarcinoma is usually peripheral • Squamous cell carcinoma is usually central.

▶ **CT findings**

Solid intrapulmonary mass of variable size; margins may be lobulated or spiculated • Central necrosis occurs in squamous cell carcinoma • Adenocarcinoma shows lesser density (ground-glass pattern) • Peritumoral lymphangitis and/or pulmonary metastases may be present • Adenocarcinoma may occur in three forms (peripheral solitary, multilocular, pneumonia-like consolidation).

▶ **MRI**

More sensitive in detecting chest wall, plexus, or mediastinal involvement • Can exclude brain metastases.

▶ **PET**

FDG-PET is the modality of choice for N and M staging (except for adenocarcinoma, where 30% false-negative findings occur) • MIBG-PET is used for tumors with neuroendocrine differentiation.

▶ **Pathognomonic findings**

Spiculated nodule with or without hilar and mediastinal lymphomas.

▶ **Diagnostic steps in nonsmall cell lung cancer**

Confirm diagnosis by imaging studies and histologic examination • Exclude distant metastases • Determine resectability.

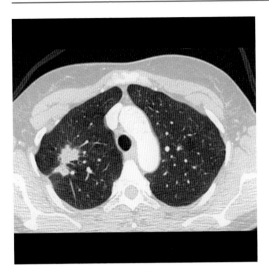

Fig. 8.1 Peripheral bronchial carcinoma (large cell carcinoma) in a 45-year-old woman. The CT shows the spiculation clearly. It also shows isolated streaky densities consistent with a fingerlike pleural lesion or microatelectasis. Findings are almost pathognomonic for a peripheral bronchial carcinoma.

Clinical Aspects

▶ **Typical presentation**
Cough ● Hemoptysis ● Dyspnea ● Chest pain.

▶ **Therapeutic options**
– *Circumscribed local tumor (stages I and II):* Surgery with or without adjuvant chemotherapy.
– *Locally advanced tumor (stage III):* Combined radiation and chemotherapy or neoadjuvant multimodal therapy concepts.
– *Stage IV (M1 with malignant pleural effusion):* Palliative chemotherapy or, where indicated, palliative radiation therapy.

▶ **Course and prognosis**
Five-year survival rate is about 10%, depending on the stage (stage Ia 75–80%, stage IIIb 5%) ● The slow-growing bronchioalveolar adenocarcinoma generally has a better prognosis.

▶ **What does the clinician want to know?**
Staging ● Complications ● Monitoring treatment.

Staging

▶ **TNM classification**
– *T staging:* T1 = Tumor diameter less than 3 cm without involvement of the main bronchus (intrapulmonary tumor) ● T2 = Tumor diameter greater than 3 cm with invasion of the main bronchus 2 cm distal to the carina, invasion of visceral pleura, or partial atelectasis or obstructive pneumonitis ● T3 = Tumor diameter greater than 7 cm with invasion of the chest wall, diaphragm, pericardium,

Fig. 8.2 Peripheral bronchial carcinoma (noncornified squamous cell carcinoma, nonsmall cell lung cancer) in a 69-year-old man. The plain chest radiographs show a large, relatively well-demarcated tumorous mass in the right posterior lower lobe. The radiographic morphology suggests an adenocarcinoma.

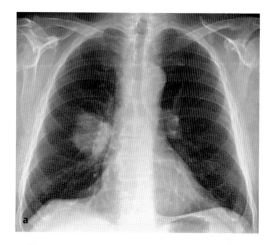

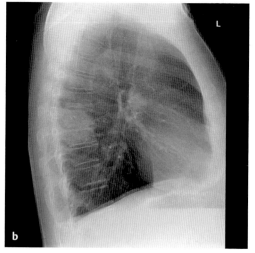

mediastinal pleura, or main bronchus adjacent to the carina (distance to the carina < 2 cm, carina free of tumor) or complete collapse of one lung or a solitary tumor node in the same lobe ● T4 = Any tumor invading the mediastinum, heart, major vessels, trachea, esophagus, spine, or carina; or separate tumor node or nodes in another ipsilateral pulmonary lobe.

– *N staging:* N1 = intrapulmonary, ipsilateral peribronchial, or ipsilateral hilar lymph nodes ● N2 = ipsilateral mediastinal and/or subcarinal lymph nodes ●

N3 = contralateral mediastinal or hilar lymph nodes, or ipsilateral or contralateral scalene or supraclavicular lymph nodes

– *M staging:* M0 = No distant metastases ● M1a = Separate tumor node or nodes on the contralateral lung, pleural nodes, or malignant pleural effusion ● M1b = Distant metastases

▶ **Stages in nonsmall cell lung cancer.**

Changes in the T categories (Goldstraw et al., 2007)

6 th edition T and M description	7th edition T and M
T1 (≤ 2 cm)	T1a
T1 (> 2–3 cm)	T1b
T2 (≤ 5 cm)	T2a
T2 (> 5–7 cm)	T2b
T2 (> 7 cm)	T3
T3 (invasion)	
T4 (same lobe nodules)	
T4 (extension)	T4
M1 (ipsilateral lung)	
T4 (pleural effusion)	M1a
M1 (contralateral lung)	M1a
M1 (distant)	M1b

Differential Diagnosis

Granuloma or tuberculoma	– Denser, more sharply demarcated, and rounder focal lesion – Calcifications – History and previous imaging studies
Hamartoma	– Asymptomatic incidental finding – Popcorn calcifications
Carcinoid	– Carcinoids, adenoid cystic carcinomas, and mucoepidermoid carcinomas primarily involve the central airways

Tips and Pitfalls

N staging based on imaging morphology is unreliable—sensitivity is about 60%, specificity about 80%, negative predictive value about 55%, and positive predictive value about 80%.

Selected References

Gilman MD, Aquino SL. State-of-the-art FDG-PET imaging of lung cancer. Semin Roentgenol 2005; 40: 143–153

Goldstraw P et al. The IASLC lung cancer staging project: proposals for the revision of the TNM stage groupings in the forthcoming (7 th) edition of the TNM classification of malignant tumors. J Thorac Oncol 2007; 2: 706–714

Mohammed TH, White CS, Pugatch RD. The imaging manifestations of lung cancer. Semin Roentgenol 2005; 40: 98–108

Ravenel JG. Lung cancer staging. Semin Roentgenol 2004; 39: 373–385

Definition

Aggressive, rapidly growing primary neoplasm of the bronchial system.

▶ **Epidemiology**
A fundamental distinction is made between small cell lung cancer (SCLC, 15–20% of cases) and nonsmall cell lung cancer (NSCLC, 80–85%) • More common in men than women • Age 40–70.

▶ **Etiology, pathophysiology, pathogenesis**
Main risk factor is cigarette smoking.

Imaging Signs

▶ **Modality of choice**
CT (including the adrenal region), PET (PET/CT) • Chest radiographs are not used in staging.

▶ **Radiographic findings**
Hilar or mediastinal mass • A pulmonary focal lesion is the exception (< 10% of cases).

▶ **CT findings**
Large mediastinal and hilar tumor with bronchial obstruction • The mass may compress major vessels (vena cava, pulmonary artery) • Obstructive atelectasis and/or pneumonitis.

▶ **MRI**
Excludes brain metastases.

▶ **PET**
FDG-PET is the modality of choice for staging (identifies disease as local or extended) • MIBG-PET identifies neuroendocrine tumors.

▶ **Pathognomonic findings**
Large mediastinal tumor involving the hilum.

▶ **Diagnostic steps in small cell lung cancer**
Confirm diagnosis by imaging studies and histologic examination • Determine stage of disease • Limited program in extended disease.

Clinical Aspects

▶ **Typical presentation**
Cough • Hemoptysis • Dyspnea • Chest pain.

▶ **Therapeutic options**
Local disease: Multimodal curative approach with surgery, chemotherapy, and radiation • *Extended disease:* Palliative chemotherapy, with adjunctive radiation therapy where indicated.

▶ **Course and prognosis**
With treatment, 5-year survival rate is 10–20% in local disease and 0–10% in extended disease.

▶ **What does the clinician want to know?**
Staging • Complications • Monitoring treatment.

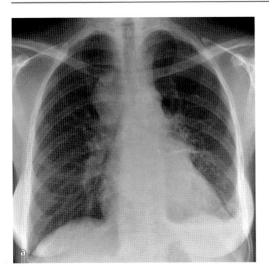

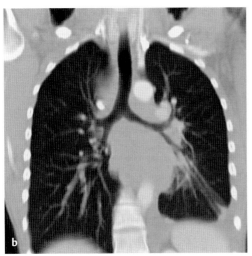

Fig. 8.3 Small cell bronchial carcinoma in a 40-year-old woman with back pain from spinal metastases.

a The plain chest radiograph shows an extensive mediastinal tumor without signs of a pulmonary lesion.

b, c On CT the findings appear as a conglomerate of lymph nodes involving all mediastinal compartments. Associated pleural effusion on the left side. The central tracheobronchial system appears normal. Only repeated bronchoscopy demonstrated the shallow tumor in the right main bronchus.

Fig. 8.3 c

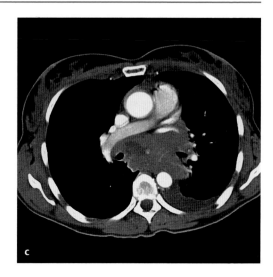

▶ **Staging**

Local disease: Tumor limited to mediastinum, hila, and supraclavicular region •
Extended disease: Extrathoracic manifestation or pulmonary metastases, malignant pleural effusion, axillary lymph node involvement.

Differential Diagnosis

Lymphoma or lymph node metastases	– Usually no signs of obstruction such as atelectasis, compression of the vena cava, or invasion or obstruction of the pulmonary artery.
Benign lymphadenopathy	– Usually smaller lymph nodes that are distinguishable from each other
Nonsmall cell lung cancer	– Pulmonary focal lesion – Fewer hilar and/or mediastinal lymph node metastases

Tips and Pitfalls

Primary site of small cell lung cancer is often unidentifiable on imaging studies.

Selected References

Gilman MD, Aquino SL. State-of-the-art FDG-PET imaging of lung cancer. Semin Roentgenol 2005; 40: 143–153

Irshad A, Ravenel JG. Imaging of small cell lung cancer. Curr Probl Diagn Radiol 2004; 33: 200–211

Definition

▶ **Epidemiology**
Variant of adenocarcinoma • 2–5% of all lung carcinomas • More common in men than in women • Peak age is about 50.

▶ **Etiology, pathophysiology, pathogenesis**
Arises from type II pneumocytes and bronchiolar epithelium • Not associated with smoking • Scarring predisposes • Spreads along the peripheral airways (bronchioloalveolar spread).

Imaging Signs

▶ **Modality of choice**
CT.

▶ **Radiographic findings**
Forms: Peripheral nodules or pneumonia-like infiltrate • Solitary (80% of cases) or multilocular to disseminated (20%).

▶ **CT findings**
– *Broad morphologic spectrum:* Peripheral nodule (ill-defined margins, lobulated or spiculated, satellite lesions) • Consolidation of a relatively low density (mucinous subtype) with CT angiogram sign, air bronchogram, and bronchiologram ("air bubbles" in 50% of cases) • Multilocular, unilateral or bilateral, disseminated appearances.
– *Density:* Solid • Ground-glass • Mixed.
– *Collateral findings:* Peripheral halo • Peritumoral lymphangitis ("crazy paving") • Peritumoral centrilobular nodules (bronchogenic spread) • Pulmonary metastases or multicentric tumors • Pleural effusion (30% of cases) • Lymphadenopathy (20%).

▶ **FDG-PET**
High rate of false-negative findings.

▶ **Pathognomonic findings**
Chronic, progressive lobar or multilobar infiltrate.

Clinical Aspects

▶ **Typical presentation**
Incidental finding in nearly asymptomatic patients, or patients may have a cough with bronchorrhea and dyspnea.

▶ **Confirmation of the diagnosis**
Bronchoalveolar lavage and transbronchial biopsy.

▶ **Therapeutic options**
Tumor resection where findings are localized • Radiation therapy and chemotherapy are indicated for nonresectable tumors.

▶ **Course and prognosis**
Prognosis is better than for other lung carcinomas due to the slow growth • Resectable tumors have a 5-year survival rate of 75%.

Fig. 8.4 Bronchioalveolar carcinoma (alveolar cell carcinoma) in a 65-year-old man.

a The plain chest radiograph shows a pneumonia-like infiltrate on the right side involving primarily the apical segments of the lower lobe and the perihilar region.

b The area of the infiltrate is hypodense on CT so that the larger vessels are delineated in addition to an air bronchogram (CT angiogram sign). Mediastinal lymphadenopathy and isolated focal infiltrates are also seen on the left side (arrows).

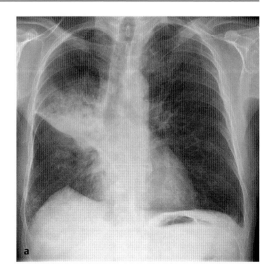

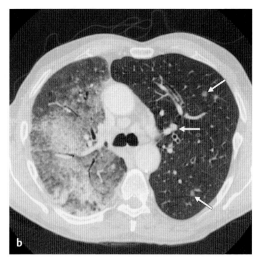

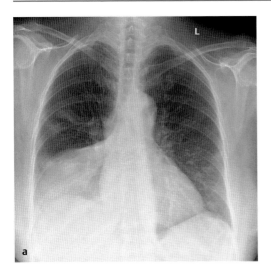

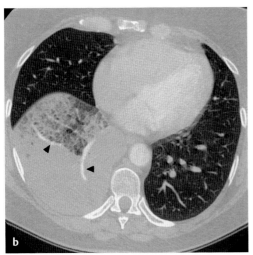

Fig. 8.5 Bronchioalveolar carcinoma (alveolar cell carcinoma) in a 60-year-old woman.

a The plain chest radiograph shows a pneumonia-like infiltrate in the right lower lobe and bilateral isolated, ill-defined focal opacities, more pronounced on the right than on the left.

b,c On CT the infiltrate appears partially as a homogeneously dense acinar shadow and partially as a less pronounced density resembling a ground-glass opacity. The CT angiogram sign (arrowhead) is prominent in both segments. The additional focal infiltrates in both lungs show a halo sign (arrows).

Fig. 8.5 c

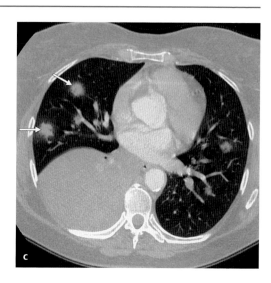

▶ **What does the clinician want to know?**
Resectability (staging as in nonsmall cell lung cancer) ● Course.

Differential Diagnosis

Peripheral bronchial carcinoma	– No air bronchogram or bronchiologram
Pneumonia	– Symptoms of infection
	– Responds to antibiotics
Cryptogenic organizing pneumonia	– Fluctuating picture
	– Responds to steroids
Wegener granulomatosis	– Renal insufficiency
	– Sinus involvement
Sarcoidosis	– Symmetrical hilar lymphadenopathy
Pulmonary lymphoma	– Usually associated with severe lymphadenopathy
Rheumatoid nodules	– Known underlying disease
Metastases	– Known underlying disease

Tips and Pitfalls

Can be misdiagnosed as chronic pneumonia.

Selected Reference

Lee KS et al. Bronchioloalveolar carcinoma: clinical, histopathologic, and radiologic findings. Radiographics 1997; 17: 1345–1357

Definition

▶ **Epidemiology**
Accounts for about 2% of all lung tumors, occurring slightly more often in women than men over a broad age range (30–60 years) • Unrelated to smoking.

▶ **Etiology, pathophysiology, pathogenesis**
Arises from neuroendocrine cells of the tracheobronchial mucosa • *Two forms:*
  – "Typical" low-grade carcinoid (80–90% of cases) • Usually occurs at a central location (main, lobar, or segmental bronchi; only rarely in the trachea) • Endoluminal or extraluminal (= "iceberg" tumor).
  – "Atypical" intermediate-grade carcinoid (10–20% of cases) • Primarily occurs at peripheral locations with or without hilar lymphadenopathy.

Imaging Signs

▶ **Modality of choice**
CT, PET/CT.

▶ **Radiographic findings**
Circumscribed, sharply demarcated hilar and/or perihilar tumor with or without obstructive atelectasis or poststenotic pneumonia (typical carcinoid), or a solitary pulmonary nodule (atypical carcinoid) • Radiographic findings are negative in 10% of cases.

▶ **CT findings**
Identical to radiographic findings • Significant contrast enhancement • Relatively specific changes occur only in a typical carcinoid at a central location—demarcation between endoluminal and extraluminal tumor components (the bronchus may be dilated) • Tumor calcification occur in about 30% of cases (less often in peripheral carcinoids) • Focal bronchiectasis with mucus retention • Lymph node metastases occur in about 10% of typical carcinoids and in about 50% of atypical carcinoids.

▶ **PET/CT findings**
Specific somatostatin receptor imaging (DOTATOC-PET/CT) has a sensitivity greater than 95%.

▶ **Pathognomonic findings**
Circumscribed, sharply demarcated hilar and/or perihilar mass with or without obstruction resulting in atelectasis, poststenotic pneumonia, and/or mucus retention.

Clinical Aspects

▶ **Typical presentation**
Cough • Hemoptysis • Recurrent pneumonia and/or atelectasis (typical carcinoid) • Cushing syndrome (ectopic ACTH syndrome) • Carcinoid syndrome with liver metastases (rare).

Fig. 8.6 Bronchial adenoma in a 32-year-old man.

a The plain chest radiograph, obtained due to recurrent respiratory distress, does not show any significant abnormal findings.

b The CT scan shows a spherical endobronchial mass in the right middle lobar bronchus, which has apparently created an intermittent valve mechanism.

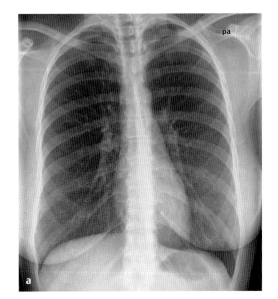

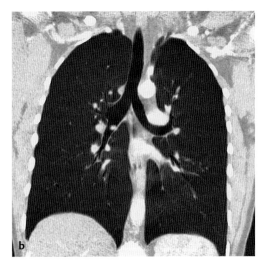

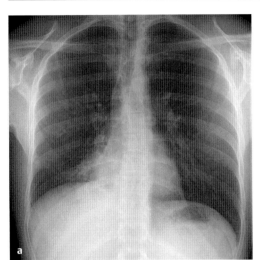

Fig. 8.7 Bronchial carcinoid in a 25-year-old man. Plain chest radiographs (**a**) were repeatedly obtained due to recurrent pulmonary infections. A lesion appearing in an identical location on several films suggested endobronchial pathology, which was confirmed by CT (**b**). The cross-sectional images show an intraluminal tumor in the right middle bronchus with infiltrates in the dependent segments.

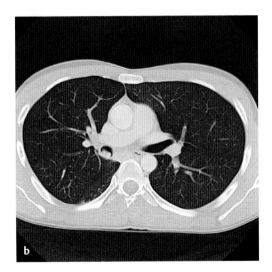

▶ **Therapeutic options**
Tumor resection.

▶ **Course and prognosis**
Typical low-grade carcinoid: 5-year survival rate is 90% without lymph node metastases ● Atypical intermediate-grade carcinoid: 5-year survival rate is 40–70%.

Differential Diagnosis

Adenoid cystic carcinoma	– Predilection for trachea and main bronchi
Mucoepidermoid carcinoma	– Indistinguishable on imaging studies
Lung carcinoma	– Associated with smoking
	– Ill-defined tumor border
	– Cavitation in squamous cell carcinoma
	– Lymphadenopathy in small cell lung cancer
	– Bubble-like air bronchiologram in adenocarcinoma
Hamartoma	– Calcification
	– Only slight contrast enhancement

Selected Reference

Jeung M et al. Bronchial carcinoid tumors of the thorax: Spectrum of radiologic findings.
Radiographics 2002; 22: 351–365

Definition

▶ **Epidemiology**
Rare ● No sex predilection ● Occurs in adults.
▶ **Etiology, pathophysiology, pathogenesis**
Benign tumorlike malformation of mixed matrix with alternating components of cartilage, bronchial epithelium, fat, and cysts.

Imaging Signs

▶ **Modality of choice**
Radiographs, CT.
▶ **Radiographic findings**
Solitary, smoothly demarcated, round, lobulated, or notched lesion of variable size (usually < 4 cm) without reaction in adjacent tissue ● Usually peripheral (90% of lesions, very rarely endobronchial) ● About 15% of lesions show popcorn calcifications.
▶ **CT findings**
Findings are identical to radiography ● CT is more sensitive in detecting cartilage calcifications and fatty components.
▶ **Pathognomonic findings**
Smoothly demarcated nodular mass with popcorn calcifications and without reaction in adjacent tissue.

Clinical Aspects

▶ **Typical presentation**
Asymptomatic incidental finding except for the very rare endobronchial hamartoma.
▶ **Confirmation of the diagnosis**
In the presence of the typical constellation of findings with popcorn calcifications and/or fatty components radiography is diagnostic, otherwise diagnosis is confirmed by biopsy or after resection.
▶ **Therapeutic options**
Resection.
▶ **Course and prognosis**
Very slow growth ● Prognosis is good ● Resection is curative.
▶ **What does the clinician want to know?**
Determine whether findings appear malignant ● Diagnosis.

Differential Diagnosis

Tuberculoma	– No popcorn calcifications
Metastasis	– Rarely solitary
	– No calcifications except osteosarcoma or in patients after chemotherapy

Fig. 8.8 Pulmonary hamartoma in a 69-year-old man (incidental finding). The plain chest radiograph (**a**) and the CT (**b**) show a sharply demarcated nodule without any reaction in adjacent tissue in the right paracardiac region. CT demonstrates fat-equivalent components but no calcifications. Biopsy confirmed the tentative diagnosis of hamartoma.

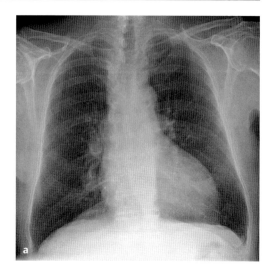

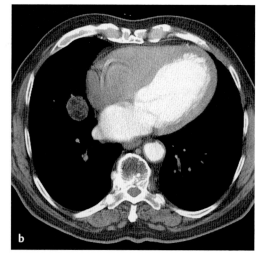

Adenocarcinoma

– In the absence of typical calcifications, hamartoma is radiographically indistinguishable from adenocarcinoma

Selected Reference

Siegelman SS et al. Pulmonary hamartoma: CT findings. Radiology 1986; 160: 313–317

Definition

Lymphoma limited to the chest and lungs, with or without mediastinal lymphadenopathy ● No extrathoracic manifestation for at least 3 months.

▶ **Epidemiology**
Rare compared with secondary lymphoma arising via hematogenous dissemination or by direct extension from hilar or mediastinal lymphomas.

▶ **Etiology, pathophysiology, pathogenesis**
Forms:
- In combination with intrathoracic lymphadenopathy ● 10–15% of lymphomas ● More common in Hodgkin disease than in non-Hodgkin lymphoma.
- Primary pulmonary lymphoma (at most with minimal lymph node involvement) ● Rare, < 1% of all malignant lymphomas ● Either Hodgkin or non-Hodgkin lymphoma ● In primary pulmonary non-Hodgkin lymphoma, a distinction is made between low-grade MALT B-cell lymphoma, high-grade non-Hodgkin lymphoma of B-cell type (about two-thirds of cases, usually associated with Epstein–Barr virus; risk groups—HIV-infected patients and organ transplant recipients), and the angioimmunoblastic lymphomas of T-cell type.

Imaging Signs

▶ **Modality of choice**
CT is preferable to plain radiography.

▶ **Radiographic findings**
Broad spectrum of findings ranging from miliary foci to nodules, pneumonia-like infiltrates (with or without air bronchogram), and interstitial and even ground-glass changes.

▶ **CT findings**
Broad spectrum of findings (in two-thirds of cases there are bilateral and/or multiple foci)—one or more nodules with or without cavitation ● Round or segmental infiltrates (with or without an air bronchogram) ● Up to 50% of high-grade lymphomas include liquefaction that may be rapidly progressive ● Reticulonodular changes.

▶ **Pathognomonic findings**
Rapidly progressive consolidations with an air bronchogram and elongated bronchovascular structures (CT angiogram sign).

Clinical Aspects

▶ **Typical presentation**
Low-grade lymphoma: Asymptomatic in > 50% of cases, otherwise mild nonspecific symptoms (cough, slight dyspnea, chest pain) ● *High-grade lymphoma:* Generally symptomatic (symptoms of hepatitis B infection).

▶ **Confirmation of the diagnosis**
Biopsy.

Fig. 8.9 Highly malignant Epstein–Barr virus-associated B-cell non-Hodgkin lymphoma in a 39-year-old man with HIV infection. Two-week history of fever, nonproductive cough, and rapid deterioration of general health.

a The plain chest radiograph shows an extensive, relatively homogeneous infiltration of the right lower lobe, enclosing a small radiolucency consistent with liquefaction.

b On CT (coronal MIP slices) the finding also appears relatively homogeneous. The major vessels and bronchi are intact (CT angiogram sign and air bronchogram).

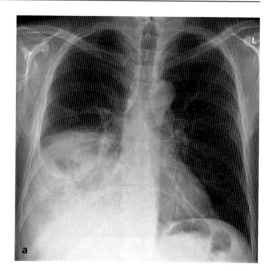

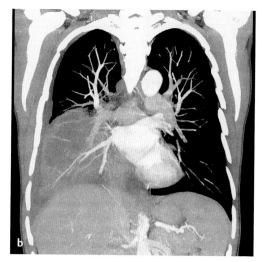

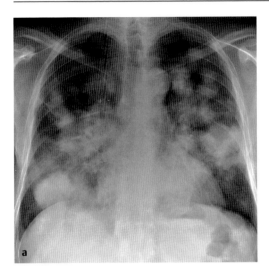

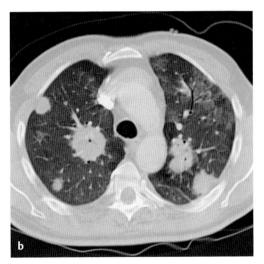

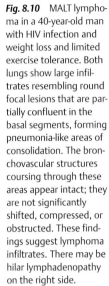

Fig. 8.10 MALT lymphoma in a 40-year-old man with HIV infection and weight loss and limited exercise tolerance. Both lungs show large infiltrates resembling round focal lesions that are partially confluent in the basal segments, forming pneumonia-like areas of consolidation. The bronchovascular structures coursing through these areas appear intact; they are not significantly shifted, compressed, or obstructed. These findings suggest lymphoma infiltrates. There may be hilar lymphadenopathy on the right side.

▶ **Therapeutic options**
Low-grade lymphoma: Watch and wait, resection, or single-modality therapy ●
High-grade lymphoma: Treatment depends on the underlying disorder, chemotherapy, modulation of immunosuppression.

▶ **Course and prognosis**
Low-grade lymphoma has a good prognosis (5-year survival rate is over 80%) ●
High-grade lymphoma has a poor prognosis, depending on the initial situation (HIV infection, organ transplantation).

▶ **What does the clinician want to know?**
Staging after diagnosis by biopsy.

Differential Diagnosis

Nodular lesions	– Bronchial neoplasm
	– Metastases
Areas of consolidation	– Pneumonia
	– Distinguished by history, clinical findings, and course
Interstitial changes	– Pulmonary interstitial disorder
Kaposi sarcoma	– Radiographically indistinguishable

Tips and Pitfalls

Because pulmonary lymphomas are rare, radiographic findings may variously be misinterpreted as pneumonia, malignancy (lung carcinoma, metastases), or pulmonary interstitial disease.

Selected References

Cadranel J, Wislez M. Antoine M. Primary pulmonary lymphoma. Eur Respir J 2002; 20: 750–762

Gimenez A et al. Unusual primary lung tumors: a radiologic-pathologic overview. Radiographics 2002; 22: 609–619

Lee DK et al. B-cell lymphoma of bronchus-associated lymphoid tissue (BALT): CT features in 10 patients. J Comput Assist Tomogr 2000; 24: 30–34

Definition

Pulmonary manifestation of juvenile laryngeal papillomatosis • Pneumatoceles due to bronchial obstruction by papilloma.

▶ **Epidemiology**
  Laryngeal papillomatosis is a common benign neoplastic disorder in children • Usually remits spontaneously during puberty • Airways distal to the larynx are involved in less than 10% of cases, the lungs in less than 1% (invasive papillomatosis).

▶ **Etiology, pathophysiology, pathogenesis**
  Viral disorder (papillomaviruses) with laryngeal and tracheobronchial manifestations secondary to perinatal infection in newborns • Solid or cystic squamous papillomas • Involvement of tracheobronchial system leads to obstructive ventilation defects.

Imaging Signs

▶ **Modality of choice**
  Radiographs, CT.

▶ **Radiographic and CT findings**
  Solid and/or cystic nodules • Diameter 1–3 cm • Minimal growth • CT shows gravitational distribution of the lesions and demonstrates intraluminal papillomas of the appropriate size (thin-slice CT) • Atelectatic areas, hyperinflated areas, and secondary bronchiectasis are rare • Fluid shadows are a sign of secondary complications.

▶ **Pathognomonic findings**
  Gravitational distribution of solid or cystic nodules.

Clinical Aspects

▶ **Typical presentation**
  Usually asymptomatic or minimally symptomatic.

▶ **Therapeutic options**
  Watch and wait strategy, as disorder is self-limiting • Antiviral or immunomodulatory therapy where indicated • Laser ablation of laryngeal and central papillomas.

▶ **Course and prognosis**
  Benign • Endoscopic intervention involves a risk of bronchopulmonary spread • Risk of malignancy is 2% (squamous cell carcinoma).

▶ **What does the clinician want to know?**
  Extent of disease • Complications.

Fig. 8.11 Known laryngeal papillomatosis with pulmonary involvement in a 17-year-old boy.

a The plain chest radiograph shows discrete cystic bullous formations which are clearly visible only in a left paracardiac location projected on the hilar region.

b CT reveals multilocular cystic lesions in both lungs, some clearly in contact with the bronchus.

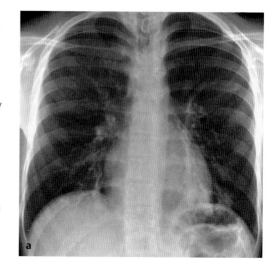

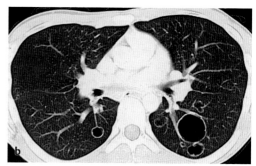

Differential Diagnosis

Pulmonary cysts	– Solitary – Thin-walled
Pneumatoceles	– Usually a temporary finding secondary to trauma or infection (see history)
Metastases	– Cystic metastases in squamous cell carcinoma and sarcoma – Growth tendency – History of known malignancy
Wegener granulomatosis	– Involvement of paranasal sinuses and kidneys
Cystic fibrosis	– Bronchiectasis with mucus retention and fluid shadows – Known underlying disease
Langerhans cell histiocytosis	– Lesions show predilection for the upper and middle lung fields – No airway involvement
Lymphangioleiomyomatosis	– Cystic lesions only – Generalized – Pleural effusion – No airway involvement – Occurs almost exclusively in women of child-bearing age

Selected References

Blackledge FA, Anand VK. Tracheobronchial extension of recurrent respiratory papillomatosis. Ann Otol Rhinol Laryngol 2000; 109: 812–818

Kawanami T, Bowen A. Juvenile laryngeal papillomatosis with pulmonary parenchymal spread. Case report and review of the literature. Pediatr Radiol 1985; 15: 102–104

Kramer SS et al. Pulmonary manifestations of juvenile laryngotracheal papillomatosis. AJR Am J Roentgenol 1985; 144: 687–694

Definition

▶ **Epidemiology**
Tumor of the apical lung characterized by arm and shoulder pain, superior sulcus tumor • Accounts for less than 5% of lung tumors.
▶ **Etiology, pathophysiology, pathogenesis**
50% squamous cell carcinomas • 25% adenocarcinomas.

Imaging Signs

▶ **Modality of choice**
MRI is preferable to CT.
▶ **Radiographic findings**
Density at the apex of the lung (apical rib companion shadow similar to a broad apical pleural cap) • Convexity is suggestive of tumor • Rib destruction (occurring in about 30% of cases) is diagnostic.
▶ **CT findings**
Tumor in the lung apex isodense to soft tissue and infiltrating the chest wall (plexus, vascular structures, ribs, spine).
▶ **MRI**
Superior to CT in demonstrating infiltration of soft tissue and the chest wall with neurovascular involvement.
▶ **PET/CT**
Superior to the other modalities in N and M staging.
▶ **Pathognomonic findings**
Mass in the apex of the lung with rib destruction.

Clinical Aspects

▶ **Typical presentation**
Unilateral shoulder pain radiating into the arm and back (90% of cases) • Horner syndrome (ptosis, miosis, and enophthalmos in 25–50% of cases).
▶ **Therapeutic options**
Neoadjuvant combined radiation and chemotherapy and en-bloc resection.
▶ **Course and prognosis**
Most cases are T3 or T4 tumors with poor prognosis • 5-year survival rate is about 15%.
▶ **What does the clinician want to know?**
Staging • Resectability.

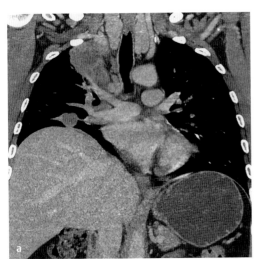

Fig. 8.12 Pancoast tumor in a 43-year-old man. The coronal (**a**) and sagittal (**b**) CT slices show a large tumor in the apex of the right lung infiltrating the mediastinum and involving the phrenic nerve. This is evidenced by the high-riding ipsilateral diaphragmatic crus. The tumor has broad contact with the pleura.

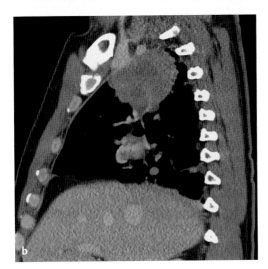

Differential Diagnosis

Radiation-induced fibrosis	– History of irradiation of the supraclavicular lymph drainage tract
Neurinoma, neurofibroma, or lateral thoracic meningocele	– Different location: paravertebral region or posterior mediastinum – Known neurofibromatosis
Aneurysm of the subclavian artery	– Readily distinguishable on ultrasound, CTA, or MRA

Tips and Pitfalls

Can be misinterpreted as an asymmetric apical pleural cap.

Selected References

Archie VC, Thomas CR. Superior sulcus tumors: a mini-review. Oncologist 2004; 9: 550–555

Jett JR. Superior sulcus tumors in Pancoast's syndrome. Lung Cancer 2003; 42 Suppl. 2: 17–21

Definition

▶ **Epidemiology**

Pulmonary metastases are common • Primary tumors in order of frequency of metastases to lung are: breast carcinoma, renal cell carcinoma, head and neck tumors, colorectal carcinoma • Frequency of pulmonary metastases according to type of primary tumor: renal cell carcinoma 75% of cases, osteosarcoma 75%, choriocarcinoma 75%, thyroid carcinoma 65%, melanoma 60%, breast carcinoma 55%.

▶ **Etiology, pathophysiology, pathogenesis**

Most lesions result from hematogenous spread (via pulmonary arteries, far less often via bronchial arteries), less often from lymphatic spread, or from pulmonary or hilar lymph node metastases.

Imaging Signs

▶ **Modality of choice**

CT is greatly preferable to plain radiography.

▶ **Radiographic and CT findings**

– Hematogenous spread usually results in multiple bilateral metastases (75% of cases) • Metastases follow the pattern of perfusion, and are more often basal than apical, more often peripheral and subpleural rather than central • Solitary metastases occur especially with colon carcinoma and renal cell carcinoma • Typically there are more or less sharply demarcated nodules of variable size, less often lobulated or ill-defined lesions (with a halo of lesser density due to perifocal hemorrhage) • Additional findings may include a feeding vessel sign; "miliary" metastases from thyroid carcinoma, melanoma, or sarcoma; liquefaction and/or cavitation (4% of cases), more common in squamous cell carcinoma than adenocarcinoma; calcifications in osteosarcoma or chondrosarcoma, papillary thyroid carcinoma, and mucinous adenocarcinoma.

– Lymphatic spread produces irregular nodular thickening of the interlobular and intralobular septa and the peribronchovascular interstitium (focal peribronchial cuffing) • Perilymphatic nodules are present • In 50% of cases they are focal, asymmetric, or unilateral.

▶ **Pathognomonic findings**

Hematogenous spread: Bilateral, predominantly basal nodules of variable size • *Lymphangitis carcinomatosa:* Inhomogeneous pattern of nodular septal and peribronchovascular thickening.

Fig. 8.13 Pulmonary metastases in a 70-year-old man with urothelial carcinoma. "Typical" findings of pulmonary metastases. Both lungs show smoothly demarcated nodules of varying size and isodense to soft tissue.

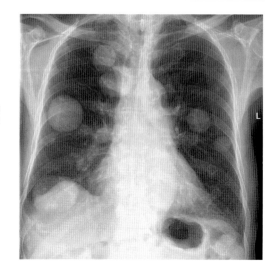

Fig. 8.14 Pulmonary metastases in a 63-year-old woman with medullary thyroid carcinoma. Both lungs are covered with small sharply demarcated nodules of nearly uniform size, creating an almost miliary picture.

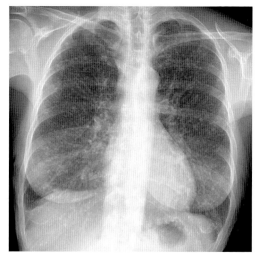

Clinical Aspects

▶ **Typical presentation**
Usually only advanced disease is symptomatic • Cough • Dyspnea • Hemoptysis.
▶ **Therapeutic options**
Pulmonary metastatic disease occurs in the setting of systemic tumor dissemination; local therapy is therefore not sufficient • Treatment depends on the underlying disorder and may include surgery, chemotherapy, radiation therapy, and/or multimodal therapy.
▶ **Course and prognosis**
Depend on the type and stage of the primary tumor.

Differential Diagnosis

Lung carcinoma	– Solitary
	– Irregular shape
	– Ill-defined border
	– Pleural spicules
Fungal infection	– More rapid growth
	– Ill-defined border
	– Underlying disorder predisposing to opportunistic infection
Rheumatoid nodules	– Usually solitary
	– Known underlying disease
Primary pulmonary lymphoma	– Rare
	– Morphologically indistinguishable

Tips and Pitfalls

Diagnostic problems may be expected only in the presence of atypical radiographic morphology and with solitary metastases • In the latter case, both evaluation of potential malignancy and differentiation from a primary lung carcinoma depend on the histological examination.

Selected References

Diederich S et al. Helical CT of pulmonary nodules in patients with extrathoracic malignancy: CT-surgical correlation. AJR Am J Roentgenol 1999; 172: 353–360

Dodd JD, Souza CA, Müller NL. High-resolution MDCT of pulmonary septic embolism: evaluation of the feeding vessel sign. AJR Am J Roentgenol 2006; 187: 623–629

Jeong YJ et al. Solitary pulmonary nodule: characterization with combined wash-in and washout features at dynamic multi-detector row CT. Radiology 2005; 237: 675–683

Quint LE, Park CH, Iannettoni MD. Solitary pulmonary nodules in patients with extrapulmonary neoplasms. Radiology 2000; 217: 257–261

Definition

Lymphatic permeation by tumor cells.

▶ **Epidemiology**
Arises from breast, lung, gastric, pancreatic, or other carcinoma (typically adeno-carcinoma).

▶ **Etiology, pathophysiology, pathogenesis**
Results from hematogenous or lymphatic spread (bronchial carcinoma, lymphoma) ● Bronchial carcinoma usually produces unilateral disease, extrathoracic primary tumor bilateral disease.

Imaging Signs

▶ **Modality of choice**
CT is preferable to plain radiography.

▶ **Radiographic findings**
Low sensitivity ● Severe cases show reticulonodular shadowing ● Septal lines ● Pleural effusion ● Lymphadenopathy.

▶ **CT findings**
Thickened interlobular septa showing a nodular or "string of pearls" pattern ● Pleural effusion (50% of cases) ● Lymphadenopathy (30%) ● Predilection for the perihilar and basal region, more often in the central interstitium than peripheral interstitium.

▶ **Pathognomonic findings**
Thickened interlobular septa showing a nodular or "string of pearls" pattern with associated pleural effusion.

Clinical Aspects

▶ **Typical presentation**
Nonproductive cough ● Initially insidious but progressive dyspnea ● Rarely the primary manifestation of malignant disease.

▶ **Therapeutic options**
Chemotherapy as indicated for the primary tumor.

▶ **Course and prognosis**
Prognosis is not favorable ● Median survival time is a matter of months.

▶ **What does the clinician want to know?**
Diagnosis or confirmation of the tentative diagnosis.

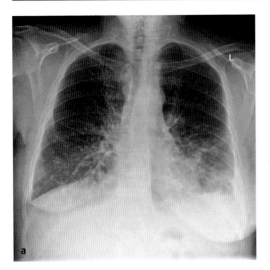

Fig. 8.15 Mixed lymphatic and hematogenous metastatic spread in a 57-year-old woman with breast carcinoma.

a The plain chest radiograph shows bronchovascular shadowing in the perihilar area and especially pronounced in lower lung fields. Other findings include an associated bilateral basal effusion.

b On CT this correlates with nodular thickened interstitial structures (arrows) and nodular deposits along the bronchovascular structures. Other findings include isolated nodules consistent with hematogenous metastases.

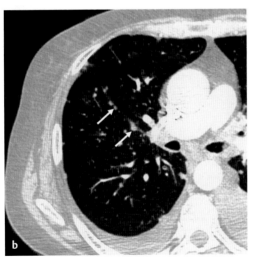

Differential Diagnosis

Interstitial pulmonary edema	– Uniformly thickened interlobular septa
	– Ground-glass opacification in dependent regions
	– Pleural effusion
Idiopathic pulmonary fibrosis	– Interstitial structures show no nodular thickening
	– Basal and subpleural distribution
	– No pleural effusion
	– No lymphadenopathy
Sarcoidosis	– Nodules independent of reticular structures
	– No pleural effusion
Scleroderma	– Linear, non-nodular interstitial structures
	– Bilateral basal distribution
	– Esophageal dilation

Tips and Pitfalls

False-negative findings are possible. Otherwise the diagnosis is usually straightforward in the context of the clinical findings.

Selected Reference

Castaner E et al. Diseases affecting the peribronchovascular interstitium: CT findings and pathologic correlation. Curr Probl Diagn Radiol 2005; 34: 63–75

Definition

▶ **Epidemiology**
Common diagnostic problem ● About half of all resected nodules are benign.
▶ **Etiology, pathophysiology, pathogenesis**
Broad etiologic spectrum: Granulomas ● Benign tumors ● Malignant tumors.

Imaging Signs

▶ **Modality of choice**
CT, PET/CT.
▶ **Radiographs, CT, and PET**
In determining whether a malignancy is present and deciding on the further diagnostic procedure, it is important to consider demographic data, history of smoking or tumor, and comorbidity in addition to the symptoms.

Criterion	Probably benign	Probably malignant Suspected malignancy
Size	< 2 cm usually benign (80%); only 1% of nodules > 5 mm are malignant	> 3 cm 25% of malignant nodules < 1 cm 42% of malignant nodules < 2 cm
Margin	Smooth (25% of benign nodules have a lobulated contour)	Irregular, lobulated, spiculated (20% of malignant nodules are smooth)
Density	< 20 HU benign > 160 HU granuloma > 200 HU calcified	Solid, semi-solid, or ground-glass (20–100 HU) potentially malignant
Calcification	Central, layered, or diffuse = granuloma Popcorn = hamartoma (One-third of noncalcified lesions on the chest radiograph show calcification on CT)	CT: amorphous, eccentric, under 10% of nodule volume (lung carcinoma, carcinoid) Radiograph: coarse calcifications in osteosarcoma
Fat	Benign (hamartoma, lipoma)	No
Contrast enhancement	Slow < 15 HU	Rapid > 20 HU
Cavitation wall	< 5 mm	> 15 mm
Growth behavior	Doubling time: < 30 or > 450 days usually benign Constant size over 2 years	Doubling time between 30 and 450 days requires evaluation
FDG-PET findings	Negative (false negative: adenocarcinoma, nodules < 7 mm)	Positive (false positive: inflammatory granulomas, anthracosis)

Fig. 8.16 Solitary pulmonary nodule in a 48-year-old man (incidental finding). The plain chest radiograph shows a sharply demarcated nodule without any reaction in adjacent tissue in the left middle lung field. CT did not demonstrate any calcifications or fat-equivalent components. Biopsy identified the lesion as a hamartoma.

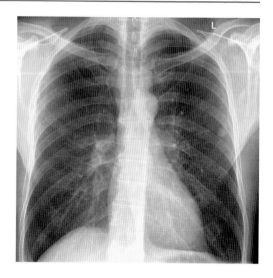

▶ **Pathognomonic findings**
Hamartoma and chondrohamartoma: Popcorn calcification and/or fatty component ● *Tuberculoma:* Central compact or layered calcification ● *Arteriovenous malformation:* Feeding and draining vessels ● *Round atelectasis:* Subpleural mass with comet tail ● *Mycetoma:* Air crescent sign ● Intrapulmonary lymph node: < 15 mm, smooth margin, oval or triangular, adjacent to the pleura or interlobar fissure.

Clinical Aspects

▶ **Typical presentation**
Usually asymptomatic incidental finding.
▶ **Therapeutic options**
Depend on the individual patient and on whether the lesion appears malignant.
▶ **Course and prognosis**
Depend on the etiology and/or underlying disorder.
▶ **What does the clinician want to know?**
Determine whether findings appear malignant ● Diagnostic options ● CT-guided biopsy.

Differential Diagnosis

Granulomas	– Postinfectious – Tuberculosis, sarcoidosis, rheumatoid nodules, or similar findings
Benign tumors	– Hamartoma, chondroma, pseudotumor
Malignant tumors	– Bronchial carcinoma, metastasis, carcinoid, Kaposi sarcoma, lymphoma
Pseudolesions	– Cutaneous changes (such as nipple shadow) – Summation phenomena

Tips and Pitfalls

Results of CAD studies show that 25% of nodules are missed ● Only 50% of the lesions seen on chest radiographs are actually singular.

Selected References

Diederich S, Hansen J, Wormanns D. Resolving small pulmonary nodules: CT features. Eur Radiol 2005; 15: 2064–2069

Erasmus JJ et al. Solitary pulmonary nodules: Part I & II. Radiographics 2000; 20: 43–58, 59–66

Leef JL, Klein JS. The solitary pulmonary nodule. Radiol Clin North Am 2002; 40: 123–143

Swenson SJ et al. Lung nodule enhancement on CT: multicenter study. Radiology 2000; 214: 73

Definition

Thrombotic occlusion of the pulmonary arterial system.

▶ **Epidemiology**
Common cause of acute chest pain with respiratory distress ● In 80% of cases however, acute pulmonary embolism remains asymptomatic.

▶ **Etiology, pathophysiology, pathogenesis**
Usually originating in the pelvic or leg veins, the thrombi restrict the blood supply to the lung ● This leads to capillary damage, transudation, hemorrhage, and occasionally necrosis.

Imaging Signs

▶ **Modality of choice**
CTA and, to a lesser extent, ventilation/perfusion scanning (lung scan).

▶ **Radiographic findings**
Nonspecific inconclusive findings: Platelike atelectasis ● High-riding diaphragm ● Pleural effusion ● Local oligemia (Westermark sign) ● Rarely pulmonary infarction, appearing as a wedge-shaped opacity with a pleural base.

▶ **CT findings**
Directly demonstrates embolisms in the pulmonary arterial system (filling defects).

▶ **Nuclear medicine**
Wedge-shaped perfusion defect.

▶ **Pathognomonic findings**
Intraluminal contrast filling defects ● Signs of right heart strain.

Clinical Aspects

▶ **Typical presentation**
Asymptomatic in about 80% of cases, rendering clinical diagnosis difficult ● Typical triad of chest pain, respiratory distress, and hemoptysis occurs in only about 5% ● Deep venous thrombosis in the pelvis or lower extremity is present in less than 50%.

▶ **Therapeutic options**
Anticoagulation and fibrinolysis ● A venal caval filter may be indicated in deep venous thrombosis in the pelvis or lower extremity where medical treatment is ineffective or contraindicated.

▶ **Course and prognosis**
Good with therapy ● Fatal in about 20% of cases if left untreated.

▶ **What does the clinician want to know?**
Confirm or exclude diagnosis ● Extent (unilateral or bilateral, central or peripheral).

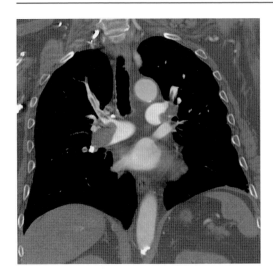

Fig. 9.1 Massive bilateral pulmonary embolism in a 79-year-old man with acute coronary syndrome. CTA shows thrombi incompletely blocking the blood flow in both main pulmonary trunks, the superior and inferior lobe arteries, and the segmental branches: findings are consistent with acute pulmonary embolism. The plain chest radiographs were normal.

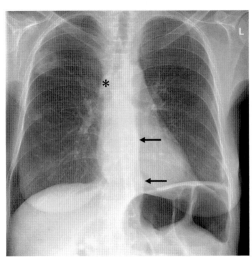

Fig. 9.2 Pulmonary infarct in a 47-year-old woman with protein S deficiency. The plain chest radiograph shows a faint wedge-shaped area of opacification with a pleural base in the right upper lung field and a second smaller area in the middle lung field consistent with infarct pneumonia. The patient had a known history of thromboembolic disease, which had led to occlusion of the inferior vena cava. Collateralization via the expanded azygos vein (∗, arrows).

Differential Diagnosis

Pneumonia	– Fever
	– One must consider the possibility of embolism where nonspecific shadows are present

Tips and Pitfalls

Insufficient filling of the pulmonary arteries • Breathing artifacts.

Selected Reference

Guilabert JP et al. Can multislice CT alone rule out reliably pulmonary embolism? A prospective study. Eur J Radiol 2007; 62: 220–226

Definition

Abnormally elevated blood pressure in the pulmonary artery (mean pulmonary arterial pressure at rest > 25 mmHg, with exercise > 30 mmHg).

▶ **Epidemiology**
Idiopathic form is rare ● Secondary forms are far more common.

▶ **Etiology, pathophysiology, pathogenesis**
Increase in pulmonary arterial pressure due to cardiac pathology (left-to-right shunt, mitral stenosis, anomalous pulmonary venous connection, etc.) or pulmonary pathology (thromboembolic disease [CTEPH], emphysema, pulmonary fibrosis, etc.) ● This leads to dilatation of the central pulmonary arteries ● Findings in idiopathic pulmonary arterial hypertension include fibrosis and proliferative muscularization of arterioles ● Pulmonary arterial hypertension is classified as idiopathic, familial, or associated; the latter occurs in disorders such as venous occlusive disease or capillary hemangiomatosis.

Imaging Signs

▶ **Modality of choice**
Radiographs, CTA, pulmonary angiography.

▶ **Radiographic findings**
Dilated central pulmonary arteries (diameter of the middle part of the right pulmonary artery > 16 mm in men, > 14 mm in women) with abrupt changes in caliber toward the periphery ● Signs of right heart strain—enlarged area of contact between the anterior wall of the heart and the sternum, prominent pulmonary trunk, prominent main pulmonary artery segment.

▶ **CTA findings**
The pulmonary trunk is wider than the ascending aorta ● Abrupt changes in caliber ● In CTEPH there are mural irregularities, intraluminal webs and bands, stenoses, and/or thromboembolic vascular occlusion ● Mosaic perfusion ● Signs of right heart strain—right ventricular dilatation and hypertrophy with protrusion of the interventricular septum against the left ventricle.

▶ **Pulmonary angiographic findings**
Vascular picture is identical to CTA.

▶ **Pathognomonic findings**
Dilated central pulmonary arteries with abrupt changes in caliber toward the periphery.

Clinical Aspects

▶ **Typical presentation**
Symptoms are nonspecific—dyspnea during exercise ● Limited exercise tolerance ● Fatigue ● Advanced-stage disease shows signs of right heart failure.

▶ **Therapeutic options**
Oxygen ● Vasodilators in primary pulmonary arterial hypertension ● Thromboendarterectomy in CTEPH ● Lung or heart–lung transplantation.

Fig. 9.3 Idiopathic pulmonary arterial hypertension in a 38-year-old woman. The plain radiograph shows signs of right heart strain with a prominent pulmonary artery segment (arrow). Prominent hila (∗) with an abrupt and severe change in caliber toward the periphery.

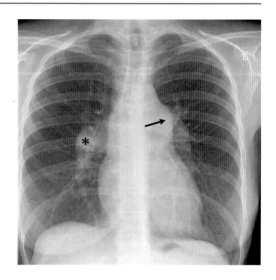

▶ **Course and prognosis**
  Poor ● 5-year survival rate in CTEPH is about 30%.
▶ **What does the clinician want to know?**
  Cause and severity of the pulmonary arterial hypertension.

Differential Diagnosis

Hilar lymphadenopathy	– More lobulated hilar mass without vascular continuity
Idiopathic pulmonary artery ectasia	– Dilation of the main pulmonary trunk and left pulmonary artery in young women without a pressure gradient
Pulmonary valve stenosis	– Dilation of the main pulmonary trunk and left pulmonary artery due to a jet effect

Tips and Pitfalls

Can be misinterpreted on the chest radiograph as lymphadenopathy.

Selected References

Coulden R. State-of-the-art imaging techniques in chronic thromboembolic pulmonary hypertension. Proc Am Thorac Soc 2006; 3: 577–583

Dorfmüller P, Humbert M, Capron F. [Vaskulopathien bei pulmonal-arterieller Hypertonie.] Pathologe 2006; 27: 140–146 [In German]

Pitton MB et al. [Chronische thrombembolische pulmonale Hypertonie: Diagnostische Wertigkeit von Mehrschicht-CT und selektiver Pulmonalis-DSA.] Fortschr Röntgenstr 2002; 174: 474–479 [In German]

Definition

▶ **Epidemiology**
Most common cause is left heart failure (coronary heart disease, myocardial infarction, cardiomyopathy, mitral valve defect).

▶ **Etiology, pathophysiology, pathogenesis**
Elevated pulmonary venous pressure (wedge pressure of 12–18 mmHg) redistributes pulmonary perfusion toward the upper lung fields (the veins cranial to the atria collapse at normal pressure) • Wedge pressure > 20 mmHg leads to edema.

Imaging Signs

▶ **Modality of choice**
Radiographs.

▶ **Radiographic findings**
The vascular structures of the upper lung fields are more pronounced (veins are more pronounced) with reflexive narrowing of the basal vessels • An abnormal heart silhouette or pleural effusion will not necessarily be present.

▶ **CT findings**
The bronchovascular bundles appear thickened, and the vessels are larger in diameter than the bronchi (normally they are of nearly equal diameter).

▶ **Pathognomonic findings**
Cranialization of pulmonary perfusion in the absence of pulmonary pathology.

Clinical Aspects

▶ **Typical presentation**
Dyspnea during physical exertion.

▶ **Therapeutic options**
Depend on the underlying cardiac disorder.

▶ **Course and prognosis**
Depend on the underlying cardiac disorder.

▶ **What does the clinician want to know?**
Congestion and/or edema.

Differential Diagnosis

Redistribution due to pulmonary pathology	– History – Abnormal pulmonary findings such as chronic obstructive pulmonary disease, emphysema, hilar pathology, etc.

Tips and Pitfalls

Can be misinterpreted as normal findings or redistribution due primarily to pulmonary pathology.

Fig. 9.4 Cardiomyopathy in a 28-year-old man. The plain chest radiograph shows widened heart silhouette with narrowing of the retrocardiac space. Significant redistribution of pulmonary perfusion toward the upper lung fields indicative of left heart failure (elevated pressure in the venous portion of the pulmonary circulation). Effusion in the left cardiophrenic angle.

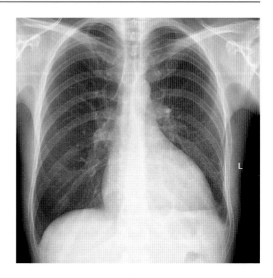

Fig. 9.5 Severe pulmonary congestion in left heart failure in a 64-year-old man. The plain chest radiograph shows generalized dilation of the heart in status post mitral stenosis, with widened and ill-defined hilar margins, and pronounced vascular structures. The widened vena cava and azygos vein are also indicative of right heart failure.

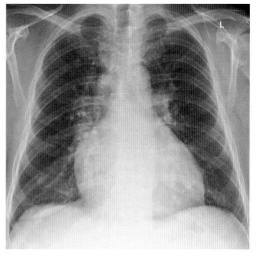

Selected References

Gehlbach BK, Geppert E. The pulmonary manifestations of left heart failure. Chest 2004; 125: 669–682

Milne ENC. Pulmonary blood flow distribution. Invest Radiol 1977; 12: 479–481

Milne ENC et al. The radiologic distinction of cardiogenic and non-cardiogenic edema. AJR Am J Roentgenol 1985; 144: 879–894

Definition

Abnormal fluid accumulation in the interstitium.

▶ **Epidemiology**

Most common cause is heart failure.

▶ **Etiology, pathophysiology, pathogenesis**

There are two pathogenetic mechanisms of pulmonary edema—hydrostatic edema and increased permeability edema ● Hydrostatic edema arises due to elevated pulmonary venous pressure in left heart disorders, obstruction of the pulmonary vein, or volume overload (hyperhydration) ● Increased permeability edema arises from increased vascular permeability as a result of alveolar and/or capillary damage or reduced osmotic pressure (oncotic edema or decreased resorption).

Imaging Signs

▶ **Modality of choice**

CT is preferable to plain radiography.

▶ **Radiographic findings**

Thickened interlobular septa (Kerley B lines) ● Blurred vascular picture ● Peribronchial cuffing ● Pleural thickening ● Decreased depth of inspiration (compliance) ● The location of the hydrostatic edema follows gravity and is usually central ● The location of the increased permeability edema follows gravity and is usually peripheral ● Associated findings in cardiogenic edema include cardiomegaly, cranialization of pulmonary perfusion, pleural effusion ● Associated findings in hyperhydration include 1 : 1 pulmonary perfusion, widened mediastinal vascular pedicle, soft tissue edema (chest wall).

▶ **CT findings**

Identical to radiographic findings ● It has higher specificity and also demonstrates posterobasal reticular shadowing.

▶ **Pathognomonic findings**

Thickened interlobular septa ● Blurred vascular picture ● Peribronchial cuffing.

Clinical Aspects

▶ **Typical presentation**

Orthopnea ● Decreased pulmonary compliance.

▶ **Therapeutic options**

Diuretics ● Oxygen ● Positive inotropic medication ● Treatment of the underlying disorder.

▶ **Course and prognosis**

Depend on the pathogenetic mechanism and underlying disorder.

▶ **What does the clinician want to know?**

Diagnosis ● Differential diagnosis ● Evaluation of severity.

Fig. 9.6 Interstitial edema in a 70-year-old woman with acute left heart failure in a hypertensive crisis. The plain chest radiograph shows prominent but blurred vascular structures due to interstitial fluid accumulation; basal interstitial shadowing, partially in the form of Kerley B lines.

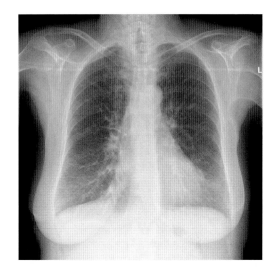

Fig. 9.7 Interstitial edema in a 76-year-old man with chronic heart failure. The plain chest radiograph shows generalized dilatation of the myopathic heart with signs of pulmonary congestion. Blurred delineation of vascular structures and increased interstitial shadowing indicative of interstitial edema.

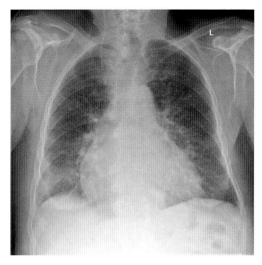

Differential Diagnosis

Interstitial pneumonia	– Fever
	– Disposition (risk patient)
	– Heart not widened
	– No pleural effusion
Lymphangitis Carcinomatosa	– History of tumor
	– Lymphadenopathy
	– Usually local
	– Normal heart silhouette

Tips and Pitfalls

Can be misinterpreted as atypical or interstitial pneumonia.

Selected References

Gluecker T et al. Clinical and radiologic features of pulmonary edema. Radiographics 1999; 19: 1507–1531

Definition

Abnormal fluid accumulation in the interstitium and alveoli.

▶ **Epidemiology**

Most common cause is heart failure.

▶ **Etiology, pathophysiology, pathogenesis**

There are two pathogenetic mechanisms of pulmonary edema—hydrostatic edema and increased permeability edema • Hydrostatic edema arises due to elevated pulmonary venous pressure in left heart disorders, obstruction of the pulmonary vein, or volume overload (hyperhydration) • Increased permeability edema arises from increased vascular permeability as a result of alveolar and/or capillary damage or reduced osmotic pressure (oncotic edema or decreased resorption).

Imaging Signs

▶ **Modality of choice**

CT is preferable to plain radiography.

▶ **Radiographic findings**

Depending on their severity and extent, findings range from ground-glass opacities to homogeneous consolidations with or without an air bronchogram • The location of the hydrostatic edema follows gravity and is usually bilateral, perihilar, and basal; "butterfly" or "bat wing" edema is rare • Location of the "toxic" increased permeability edema is usually peripheral • Associated findings in cardiogenic edema include cardiomegaly, cranialization of pulmonary perfusion, pleural effusion (usually bilateral or primarily on the right side).

▶ **CT findings**

Findings are identical to radiography.

▶ **Pathognomonic findings**

Bilateral, primarily perihilar and basal ground-glass opacities or areas of consolidation with pleural effusion in cardiogenic edema, usually peripheral location in "toxic" edema.

Clinical Aspects

▶ **Typical presentation**

Orthopnea to dyspnea, depending on severity • Foamy blood-tinged sputum • Auscultatory findings.

▶ **Therapeutic options**

Diuretics • Oxygen • Positive inotropic medication • Assisted ventilation where indicated • Treatment of the underlying disorder.

▶ **Course and prognosis**

Depend on the pathogenetic mechanism and underlying disorder.

▶ **What does the clinician want to know?**

Diagnosis • Differential diagnosis • Evaluation of severity.

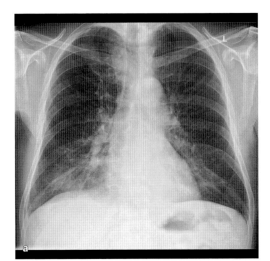

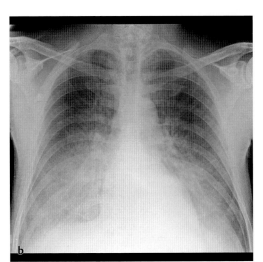

Fig. 9.8 The plain chest radiograph shows alveolar pulmonary edema in a 55-year-old man with aortic valve disease and endocarditis.

a Signs of left heart failure with vascular blurring and opacification of the mediobasal lower lung fields indicative of interstitial fluid accumulation.

b The follow-up study the next day showed increasing opacification of the lower lung fields with masking of vascular structures by the now clearly visible alveolar edema.

Differential Diagnosis

Pneumonia	– Fever
	– Usually localized infiltrates without gravitational distribution
	– Usually normal-sized heart
Pulmonary hemorrhage	– Symptoms are mild compared with radiographic findings
	– Opacities without gravitational distribution
	– Normal cardiac findings
	– No pleural effusion
Alveolar proteinosis	– Symptoms are mild compared with radiographic findings
	– Opacities without gravitational distribution
	– Normal cardiac findings
	– No pleural effusion
Adult respiratory distress syndrome	– History
	– Assisted ventilation is indicated
	– Pleural effusion is rare

Tips and Pitfalls

Can be misinterpreted as pneumonia.

Selected Reference

Gluecker T et al. Clinical and radiologic features of pulmonary edema. Radiographics 1999; 19: 1507–1531

Definition

▶ **Epidemiology**
Most common mediastinal cysts ● Developmental anomalies of the embryonal foregut ● Isolated cystic lesions ● Forms include pericardial cysts, thymic cysts, bronchogenic cysts, esophageal duplication cysts, and neuroenteric cysts.

▶ **Etiology, pathophysiology, pathogenesis**
Bronchogenic cysts arise from the ventral foregut, enteric cysts from the dorsal foregut ● Bronchogenic cysts contain respiratory epithelium, smooth muscle, and cartilage; enteric cysts contain squamous and gastrointestinal epithelium, smooth muscle, and nerve plexus.

Imaging Signs

▶ **Modality of choice**
MRI is equivalent to CT.

▶ **CT and MRI findings**
Smoothly demarcated, thin-walled, cystic, spherical or ellipsoid mass showing no enhancement with contrast ● Cysts with serous contents (most common) exhibit water-equivalent density (most common in pericardial cysts), those with other contents (mucus, calcium milk, blood) show higher density ● Bronchogenic cysts may show calcified walls ● Cysts rarely communicate with the tracheobronchial or esophageal lumen (air–fluid level) ● On MRI, cysts show variable signal behavior depending on the contents, typically appearing markedly hyperintense on T2-weighted sequences and hypointense or hyperintense on T1-weighted sequences ● Bronchogenic cysts are usually subcarinal and paratracheal (> 50% on the right side, 15% in the pulmonary region) ● Esophageal duplication cysts usually occur in a distal paraesophageal location (more often on the right than left) and are rarely intramural ● Neuroenteric cysts occur in the mediastinum superior to the carina and in 50% of cases are associated with spinal anomalies.

▶ **Pathognomonic findings**
Water-equivalent density and signal intensity ● No enhancement ● Typical location ● Neuroenteric cysts are associated with spinal anomalies.

Clinical Aspects

▶ **Typical presentation**
One-third are asymptomatic incidental findings ● Two-thirds are symptomatic (causing airway or esophageal obstruction) and usually already manifest in infancy.

▶ **Therapeutic options**
Complete surgical resection is usually indicated even for asymptomatic cysts ● Pericardial cysts usually require no treatment.

▶ **Course and prognosis**
Prognosis is excellent following complete excision.

Fig. 10.1 Pericardial cyst in a 52-year-old woman (incidental finding). The plain chest radiograph (**a**) shows a circumscribed convex shadow in the right cardiophrenic angle with a cardiac silhouette sign. The shape and location suggest a pericardial cyst. This was confirmed on MRI, where the lesion exhibited signal intensity typical of a cyst (**b**).

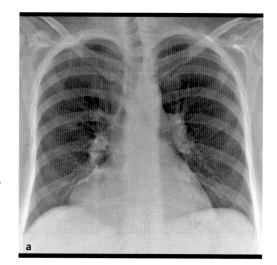

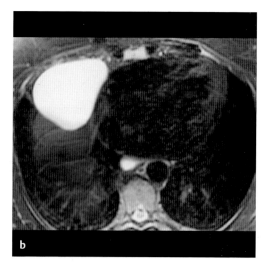

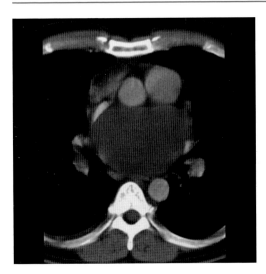

Fig. 10.2 MR image of a bronchogenic cyst. The cyst has a typical spherical shape, is smoothly demarcated, thin-walled, and exhibits homogeneous, fluid-equivalent density.

▶ **What does the clinician want to know?**
Diagnosis and differential diagnosis ● Location and extent (resection) ● Impairment of adjacent structures.

Differential Diagnosis

Thymus cyst	– Location: upper anterior mediastinum
Pericardial cyst	– Pericardial contact – Usually in the cardiophrenic angle (right side in 70% of cases, left in 22%) – Invariably water equivalent
Lymphangioma	– Occurs in infancy – Multicystic or septate – With axial or cervical ramifications
Meningocele	– Paravertebral cystic formation isodense and isointense to CSF and continuous with the dural sac – Occasionally with widening of the neural foramen
Tumor cysts	– Thymic and germ cell tumors: solid tumor components predominate
Pancreatic pseudocyst	– Signs of a complicated cyst (irregularity, septation, marginal enhancement, reaction in adjacent tissue) – History of pancreatitis

Fig. 10.3 Thymic cyst.
a The plain chest radiograph shows a widening of the mediastinal shadow on the right by a large, smoothly demarcated paracardiac mass with a shallow convex lateral margin obscuring the right margin of the heart (silhouette sign).

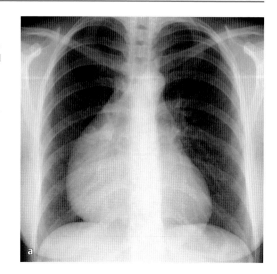

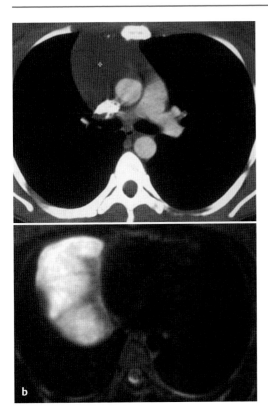

b CT (above) and MRI (below) show liquid cystic findings. The thymic cyst was confirmed intraoperatively. The size and cranial location are largely inconsistent with a pericardial cyst.

Tips and Pitfalls

Can be misdiagnosed as a solid mass ● Complicated cysts are not clearly distinguishable from cystic tumors.

Selected References

Jeung MY et al. Imaging of cystic masses of the mediastinum. Radiographics 2002; 22: 79–93

Kim JH, Goo JM, Lee HJ. Cystic tumors in the anterior mediastinum: radiologic-pathological correlation. J Comput Assist Tomogr 2003; 27: 714–723

Strollo DC, Rosado-de-Christensom ML, Jett JR. Primary mediastinal tumors: Part 1 Tumors of the anterior mediastinum. Part 2 Tumors of the middle and posterior mediastinum. Chest 1997; 112: 511–522, 1344–1357

Takeda S, Miyoshi S, Minami M. Clinical spectrum of mediastinal cysts. Chest 2003; 124: 125–132

Definition

▶ **Epidemiology**
Goiter occurs on average in about 5% of the population (in Germany), about 20% of these have an intrathoracic component ● Three times as common in women than in men.

▶ **Etiology, pathophysiology, pathogenesis**
Primary goiter occurs with an accessory intrathoracic thyroid (with thoracic vascular supply) ● Secondary goiter develops as a ramification of a cervical goiter (with cervical vascular supply) ● Develops in response to thyroid-stimulating hormone in iodine deficiency or thyroid insufficiency.

Imaging Signs

▶ **Modality of choice**
Radiographs, CT, nuclear medicine.

▶ **Radiographic findings**
Smoothly demarcated space-occupying lesion in the anterior upper mediastinum that moves when the patient swallows and leads to tracheal shift and/or compression ● Calcifications occur in 25% of cases.

▶ **CT findings**
Smoothly demarcated mass appearing hyperdense on plain scans due to iodine (70–120 HU) and located in the upper mediastinum (75% anterior to the trachea, 25% posterior) ● Tracheal shift (occasionally with compression) ● Calcifications and colloid cysts are common findings ● Enhances markedly on contrast-enhanced CT ● Contrast-enhanced CT scans should be performed only after nuclear medicine studies.

▶ **Nuclear medicine**
Nuclide uptake (iodine-123) equivalent to thyroid tissue.

▶ **Pathognomonic findings**
Mass in the anterior upper mediastinum continuous with the thyroid and displacing and/or compressing the trachea and/or esophagus.

Clinical Aspects

▶ **Typical presentation**
Usually asymptomatic where only mild hypothyroidism is present (variable thyroid function is normal; thyroid function tests are indicated) ● Stridor and/or dyspnea, dysphagia, and dysphonia depending on size and location.

▶ **Therapeutic options**
Surgical resection is indicated for large symptomatic goiters and where malignancy is suspected ● Thyroid function tests are invariably indicated.

▶ **Course and prognosis**
Prognosis is good for benign goiters ● Prognosis for malignant goiters depends on the histology.

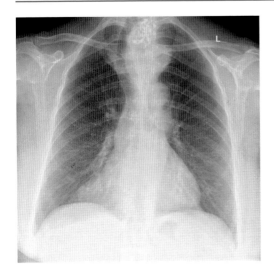

Fig. 10.4 Retrosternal goiter in a 66-year-old woman. The plain chest radiograph shows a space-occupying lesion at the level of the thoracic inlet with coarse patchy calcifications and a right convex tracheal shift. Other findings include a fatty mass in the right paracardiac region.

▶ **What does the clinician want to know?**
Confirmation of tentative diagnosis • Determine whether findings appear malignant • Thyroid function.

Differential Diagnosis

Thymic tumor	– Located farther caudally and not continuous with the thyroid – Lesser density and enhancement on CT
Teratoma	– Located farther caudally and not continuous with the thyroid – Lesser density and enhancement on CT – Fatty components
Lymphoma	– No calcifications initially – Multinodular – Lesser density and enhancement on CT
Castleman disease	– Strong contrast enhancement similar to goiter – Not continuous with the thyroid – Multinodular and multilocular

Tips and Pitfalls

Difficulties with differential diagnosis are to be expected only with the primary form.

Selected References

Duwe BV, Sterman DH, Musani AI. Tumors of the mediastinum. Chest 2005; 128: 2893–2909

Strollo DC, Rosado-de-Christenson ML, Jett JR. Primary mediastinal tumors: Part 1 Tumors of the anterior mediastinum. Chest 1997; 112: 511

Fig. 10.5 Retrosternal goiter in a 76-year-old woman. The axial (**b**) and coronal CT-images show a severe cervical goiter with regressive changes (cystic necrotic components and calcifications). The goiter extends far into the anterior upper mediastinum, significantly displacing the carotid arteries and brachiocephalic veins. The trachea shows a right convex shift with only slight compression. The cardinal diagnostic criteria are the continuity of the mediastinal mass with the thyroid and its equivalent texture.

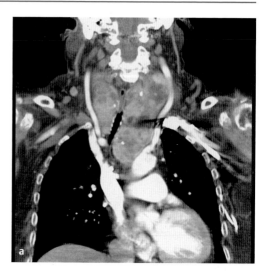

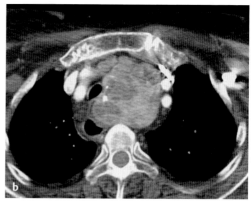

Definition

▶ **Epidemiology**
Account for about 20% of primary mediastinal tumors ● Most common mass in the anterior mediastinum aside from teratoma, lymphoma, and goiter ● Occurs exclusively in the anterior mediastinum anterior to the heart and great vessels ● Occurs at age 40–60 ● Often associated with other clinical pictures and findings (especially myasthenia gravis, red cell aplasia, hypogammaglobulinemia).

▶ **Etiology, pathophysiology, pathogenesis**
The classification of thymomas is based on the predominant cell type, epithelial or lymphocytic ● Encapsulated and invasive lymphomas are histologically identical ● Other thymic tumors and tumorlike processes include thymic cyst, thymic lipoma, thymic carcinoma, and thymic carcinoid.

Imaging Signs

▶ **Modality of choice**
CT is preferable to MRI.

▶ **CT findings**
– *Thymoma:* Solid round or oval smoothly demarcated mass in the anterior upper mediastinum (usually < 10 cm) ● Necrotic, cystic, hemorrhagic components in up to 30% of cases ● Calcifications in 25% (not a criterion of malignancy) ● 35% of thymomas show locally invasive growth—pericardial thickening, vascular encasement, pleural metastases ● Invasive forms of thymoma are indistinguishable from thymic carcinoma, thymic carcinoid, or malignant germ cell tumor.
– *Thymic carcinoma:* Usually > 10 cm ● Irregular ● Ill-defined margin ● Signs of invasion ● Heterogeneous enhancement ● Involvement of mediastinal lymph nodes in 40% of cases ● Metastases (lung, liver) in 30%.
– *Thymic cyst:* Thin-walled ● Usually a solitary finding.
– *Thymic lipoma:* Sharply demarcated ● Fat-equivalent density.
– *Thymic carcinoid:* Resembles a thymoma ● Involvement of mediastinal lymph nodes or metastases in 20–30% of cases.

▶ **MRI findings**
– *Thymoma:* Isointense to muscle on T1-weighted sequences, cystic components are hypointense ● Hyperintense on T2-weighted sequences, cystic components are markedly hyperintense.
– *Thymic carcinoma:* Heterogeneous signal behavior and enhancement.
– *Thymic cyst:* Hypointense on T1-weighted sequences ● Markedly hyperintense on T2-weighted sequences.

▶ **Pathognomonic findings**
Round or oval lobulated mass in the anterior upper mediastinum < 10 cm.

Fig. 10.6   Thymoma in a 43-year-old man. The plain chest radiograph shows a large mass in the right anterior mediastinum. On the lateral film (**b**) the tumor shows a convex partial calcification. Slightly high-riding right diaphragmatic crus. Histological examination revealed a thymoma with no evidence of malignancy.

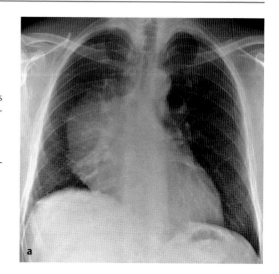

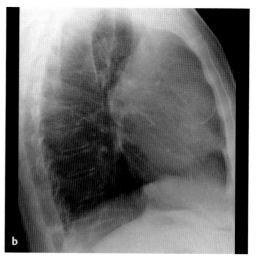

Clinical Aspects

▶ **Typical presentation**
  - *Thymoma:* Myasthenia gravis (diplopia, ptosis, weakness) in 50% of cases.
  - *Thymic carcinoma:* Chest pain ● Weight loss ● Paraneoplastic syndrome in rare cases.
  - *Thymic carcinoid:* Paraneoplastic syndrome is common (33% of cases) ● Cushing syndrome ● Multiple endocrine neoplasia (MEN) 1 syndrome.
  - *Thymic cyst and thymic lipoma:* Asymptomatic incidental findings.
▶ **Therapeutic options**
  Resection.
▶ **Course and prognosis**
  Thymoma: Prognosis is good where the capsule is intact, moderate for invasive cases ● *Thymic carcinoma:* Poor prognosis.
▶ **What does the clinician want to know?**
  Localization and extent (for biopsy and/or resection) ● Involvement of adjacent structures.

Differential Diagnosis

Retrosternal goiter	– Continuous with the thyroid
	– Higher density than muscle on CT
	– Regressive changes are common
Lymphoma	– Thymic involvement in the setting of a generalized lymphoma (usually Hodgkin disease)
Teratoma or germ cell tumors	– Similar cross-sectional morphology
	– Clinical findings and laboratory results are required to distinguish these disease entities

Tips and Pitfalls

Thymic carcinoma is indistinguishable from invasive thymoma on imaging studies ● Complete resection is required to distinguish between the two conditions.

Selected References

Duwe BV, Sterman DH, Musani AI. Tumors of the mediastinum. Chest 2005; 128: 2893–2909
Nishino M et al. Thymus—a comprehensive review. Radiographics 2006; 26: 335–348
Strollo DC, Rosado-de-Christenson ML, Jett JR. Primary mediastinal tumors: Part 2 Tumors of the middle and posterior mediastinum. Chest 1997; 112: 1344–1357

Definition

▶ **Epidemiology**
  Germ cell tumors account for about 15% of primary mediastinal tumors • Predilection for the anterior mediastinum, often adjacent to the thymus • Predilection for young men • Teratoma is the most common germ cell tumor of the mediastinum, seminoma the most common malignant form.

▶ **Etiology, pathophysiology, pathogenesis**
  The germ cell tumors include teratomas (usually benign, rarely teratocarcinomas), seminomas, and nonseminomatous germ cell tumors (embryonal carcinoma, yolk sac tumors, choriocarcinoma, and mixed tumors).

Imaging Signs

▶ **Modality of choice**
  CT, MRI.

▶ **CT and MRI findings**
  – *Seminoma:* Large solid, usually lobulated mass of homogeneous density; cystic or necrotic areas are rare
  – *Teratomas:* Mature teratomas are the only germ cell tumors to exhibit typical findings (see below)
  – *Teratocarcinoma:* Irregularly demarcated tumor with inhomogeneous contrast enhancement, calcifications, necrosis, and signs of infiltration.

▶ **Pathognomonic findings**
  Mature teratomas are the only germ cell tumors to exhibit typical findings on imaging studies—they are well demarcated round or lobulated tumors with cysts, calcifications or ossifications, and fatty tissue (50% of cases) • Primordia of tooth and/or bone or fat–fluid levels are pathognomonic findings.

Clinical Aspects

▶ **Typical presentation**
  Asymptomatic incidental finding or symptomatic lesion • Symptomatic tumors (cough, pain, dyspnea, fever) suggest malignancy • AFP is elevated in embryonal carcinomas and yolk sac tumors • HCG is elevated in choriocarcinoma • Pure seminomas do not show raised AFP and only occasionally raised HCG (10% of cases). Exclude a primary testicular tumor.

▶ **Therapeutic options**
  Mature teratomas: Resection • *Seminomas:* Combined radiation therapy and chemotherapy • *Nonseminomatous germ cell tumors:* Chemotherapy and resection.

▶ **Course and prognosis**
  Mature teratomas: Excellent prognosis • *Pure seminomas:* Very good prognosis • *Mixed tumors:* Variable prognosis.

▶ **What does the clinician want to know?**
  Localization and extent (for biopsy and/or resection) • Involvement of adjacent structures.

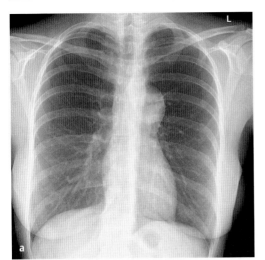

Fig. 10.7 Mature teratoma in a 37-year-old woman (incidental finding).

a The plain chest radiograph shows a sharply demarcated convex mass in the aortopulmonary window.

b CT also shows a smoothly demarcated lesion with focal mural calcifications and components isodense to fat and soft tissue.

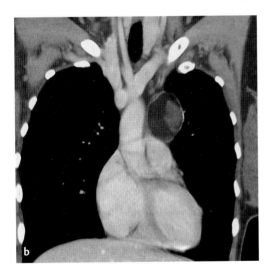

Fig. 10.8 Extragonadal germ cell tumor in a 26-year-old man with chest pain.

a The plain chest radiograph shows an abnormally widened anterior upper mediastinum.

b CT visualizes the tumor as a lobular mass with inhomogeneous density and liquid components suggestive of necrosis.

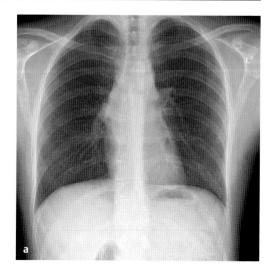

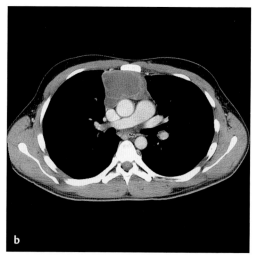

Differential Diagnosis

Lymphoma	– Homogeneous solid mass
	– Multilocular
	– Often indistinguishable from a seminoma
Thymoma or thymic tumor	– Indistinguishable from malignant germ cell tumors
Retrosternal goiter	– Continuous with the thyroid
	– Higher density than muscle on CT

Tips and Pitfalls

Except for mature teratomas, it is impossible to determine whether findings are malignant.

Selected References

Duwe BV, Sterman DH, Musani AI. Tumors of the mediastinum. Chest 2005; 128: 2893–2909

Kim JH, Goo JM, Lee HJ. Cystic tumors in the anterior mediastinum: radiologic-pathological correlation. J Comput Assist Tomogr 2003; 27: 714–723

Moeller KH, Rosado-de-Christenson ML, Templeton DA. Mediastinal mature teratoma: imaging features. AJR Am J Roentgenol 1997; 169: 985–990

Strollo DC, Rosado-de-Christenson ML, Jett JR. Primary mediastinal tumors: Part 1 Tumors of the anterior mediastinum. Chest 1997; 112: 511

Definition

▶ **Epidemiology**
Account for 10–20% of mediastinal masses ● 90% occur in the posterior mediastinum ● Usually benign (80%).

▶ **Etiology, pathophysiology, pathogenesis**
Several forms are differentiated: Peripheral nerve sheath tumors (schwannomas or neurilemmomas, neurofibromas, malignant nerve sheath tumors; usually in adults) ● Tumors of the sympathetic ganglia (ganglioneuromas, ganglioneuroblastomas, neuroblastomas; usually in children under 10) ● Tumors of the parasympathetic ganglia (very rare).

Imaging Signs

▶ **Modality of choice**
CT and MRI are indicated to evaluate intraspinal findings ● MIBG imaging in neuroblastoma.

▶ **CT findings**
– *Schwannoma and neurofibroma:* Paravertebral, smoothly demarcated round or lobulated mass isodense to soft tissue extending over one to two intercostal spaces ● Homogeneous or heterogeneous density ● Homogeneous, heterogeneous, or marginal enhancement ● In 50% of cases there is compressive excavation of the vertebrae and or ribs ● Widening of the neural foramen occurs with hourglass tumors (10%) ● Plexiform neurofibroma is a variant.
– *Ganglioneuroma and ganglioneuroblastoma:* Tumor tends to be long, extending over three to five segments with broad anterolateral contact with the spine ● Homogeneous or heterogeneous density (stippled calcifications may occur) ● Enhances moderately with contrast ● Signs of malignancy include size > 5 cm, heterogeneity, local invasiveness (mediastinum or chest wall), hematogenous metastases (lung).

▶ **MRI findings**
– *Schwannoma and neurofibroma:* Morphologic criteria as on CT ● Low to intermediate signal intensity on T1-weighted sequences, intermediate to high signal intensity on T2-weighted sequences.
– *Ganglioneuroma and ganglioneuroblastoma:* Heterogeneous signal intensity on all sequences.

▶ **Pathognomonic findings**
Smoothly demarcated round or lobulated tumors in a typical paravertebral location with compressive erosion of bone ● Multiple neurogenic tumors and plexiform neurofibromas are pathognomonic for neurofibromatosis.

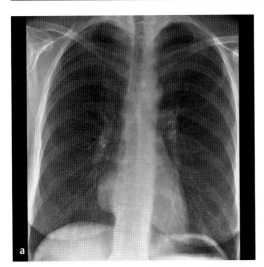

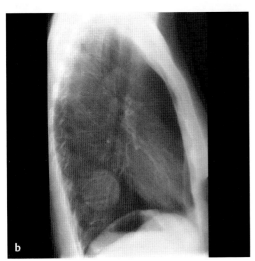

Fig. 10.9 Neurilemoma in a 48-year-old man. The plain chest radiographs show only a spherical, smoothly demarcated paravertebral mass of soft tissue density in the posterior lower mediastinum. Even without widening of the intervertebral foramen, the lesion is most likely a neurogenic tumor because of its location. The lesion was confirmed intraoperatively as a neurilemoma.

Fig. 10.10 Neurofibroma in a 38-year-old woman.

a The plain chest radiograph shows bilateral abnormal widening of the upper mediastinum primarily on the left side involving the thoracic inlet. A second tumor of soft tissue density is visualized laterally along the ribs in the left upper lung field. A local density is also visible projected on the right hilum.

b–e The CT images show the lesion in each case to be a smoothly demarcated extrapulmonary tumor homogeneously isodense to soft tissue without any bony destruction. Local widening of the intervertebral foramen was demonstrated only at the level of the thoracic inlet (not shown).

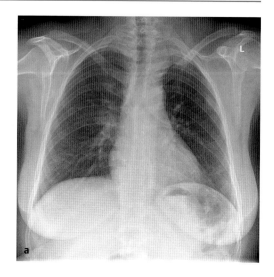

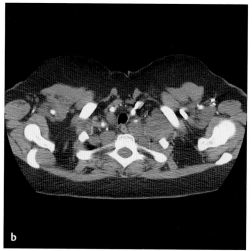

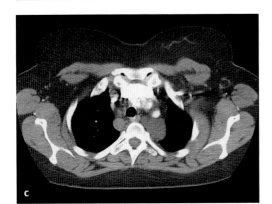

Fig. 10.10 c–e

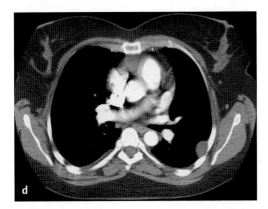

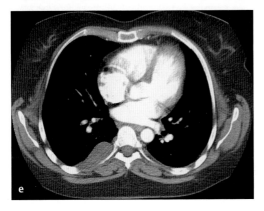

Clinical Aspects

▶ **Typical presentation**

The majority of benign tumors are asymptomatic • The majority of malignant tumors are symptomatic (pain, paresthesias, neurologic deficits) • A metabolically active neuroblastoma or ganglioneuroblastoma produces catecholamines and intestinal peptides that can cause hypertension, flush symptoms, and diarrhea.

▶ **Therapeutic options**

Radical surgical excision • Chemotherapy and resection are indicated for neuroblastoma and ganglioneuroblastoma.

▶ **Course and prognosis**

Prognosis is good for benign tumors that are excised completely • Local recurrence is common following incomplete resection or in neurofibromatosis • The prognosis for malignant tumors depends on the initial findings and the opportunity for radical treatment but on the whole is quite unfavorable.

▶ **What does the clinician want to know?**

Involvement of the spinal canal • Determine whether findings appear malignant (local invasiveness, metastases) • Staging in neuroblastoma and ganglioneuroblastoma:

Stage I: Ipsilateral, circumscribed, noninvasive

Stage II: Locally invasive, does not cross the midline, no lymph node metastases

Stage III: Crosses the midline, bilateral regional lymph node metastases

Stage IV: Extensive metastases

Stage IVS: Stage I or II tumors with metastases limited to the liver, skin, and/or bone marrow

Differential Diagnosis

Lateral thoracic meningocele	– Isodense and isointense to CSF
	– Communicates with the spinal canal
	– Asymptomatic
	– Associated with neurofibromatosis in 75% of cases
Extramedullary hemopoiesis	– Long chimneylike cuff of paravertebral soft tissue
	– Associated hepatosplenomegaly
Paraspinal abscess	– Typical abscess with broad band of marginal enhancement and central hypodensity on CT and high signal intensity on T2-weighted MRI sequences
	– Associated spondylitis
Paraspinal hematoma	– Usually posttraumatic
	– Associated spinal fracture

Tips and Pitfalls

Determine whether the lesion appears malignant.

Selected References

Forsythe A, Volpe J, Muller R. Posterior mediastinal ganglioneurinoma. Radiographics 2004; 24: 594–597

Franco A, Mody NS, Meza MP. Imaging evaluation of pediatric mediastinal masses. Radiol Clin North Am 2005; 43: 325–353

Reeder LB. Neurogenic tumors of the mediastinum. Semin Thorac Cardiovasc Surg 2000; 12: 261–267

Stark DD, Moss AA, Brasch RC. Neuroblastoma: diagnostic imaging and staging. Radiology 1983; 148: 101–105

Definition

▶ **Epidemiology**
The mediastinum is the initial site of malignant lymphoma in 10% of cases • Mediastinal involvement occurs in 50% of cases in Hodgkin disease and in 20% in non-Hodgkin lymphoma.

▶ **Etiology, pathophysiology, pathogenesis**
Hodgkin disease (especially the nodular sclerosis type) shows a predilection for the anterior mediastinum and thymus • Non-Hodgkin lymphoma (large cell B-cell lymphoma and lymphoblastic lymphomas) show a predilection for the middle and posterior mediastinum, and paracardiac and mammary lymph nodes.

Imaging Signs

▶ **Modality of choice**
CT, MRI, FDG-PET.

▶ **Radiographic findings**
Abnormal mediastinal widening occurs in 75% of cases in Hodgkin disease and < 50% in non-Hodgkin lymphoma.

▶ **CT findings**
Isolated abnormally enlarged lymph nodes or conglomerate tumor • Homogeneous density • Uniform contrast enhancement.
   – *Hodgkin disease:* Predilection for the anterior mediastinum • Pericardial effusion occurs in invasion • Pulmonary involvement occurs only with hilar lymphomas.
   – *Non-Hodgkin lymphoma:* Predilection for the middle and posterior mediastinum, paracardiac and parasternal lymph nodes. • Discontinuous dissemination • Pulmonary involvement may also occur without hilar lymphomas.

▶ **MRI findings**
Hodgkin disease and non-Hodgkin lymphoma: Hypointense on T1-weighted sequences (isointense to muscle), hyperintense or of intermediate intensity on T2-weighted sequences, hypointense where extensive fibrosis is present • Other findings are similar to CT.

▶ **FDG-PET**
Modality of choice for monitoring treatment and for staging.

▶ **Pathognomonic findings**
Massively enlarged lymph nodes of homogeneous density and signal intensity.

Clinical Aspects

▶ **Typical presentation**
   – Hodgkin disease is often a minimally symptomatic incidental finding (pain, dyspnea, dysphagia) • Fever, night sweats, and weight loss occur in 25% of cases • Superior vena cava syndrome is rare.

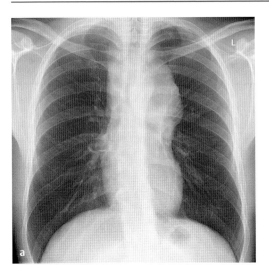

Fig. 10.11 Hodgkin disease. The plain chest radiograph (**a**) shows chimneylike widening of the upper mediastinum with a polycyclic contour on the left side. The aortic knob and descending aorta are distinguishable, which suggests a mass in the anterior mediastinum. The lateral film (**b**) confirms this.

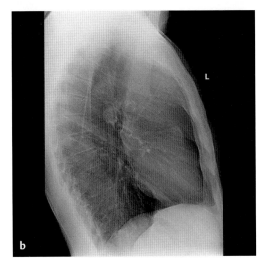

– Non-Hodgkin lymphoma is symptomatic in 85% of cases (generalized symptoms, generalized lymphadenopathy) • Large cell B-cell lymphoma and lymphoblastic lymphoma initially manifest in the anterior mediastinum in young patients as a rapidly progressive mediastinal tumor with acute or subacute symptoms (shortness of breath and superior vena cava syndrome).

▶ **Therapeutic options**
- *Hodgkin disease:* Stage I or II is treated with radiation therapy ● Stage III or IV, chemotherapy or combined radiation and chemotherapy.
- *Non-Hodgkin lymphoma:* Treated with aggressive chemotherapy or combined radiation and chemotherapy and bone marrow transplantation.

▶ **Course and prognosis**
- *Hodgkin disease:* Prognosis depends on the stage ● Cure rates for stages IA and IIA > 90%, stage IV 50%.
- *Non-Hodgkin lymphoma:* Prognosis depends primarily on the histology ● Negative prognostic factors include tumor volume, extranodal dissemination, poor response to treatment.

▶ **What does the clinician want to know?**
Confirmation of tentative diagnosis ● Staging of Hodgkin disease:

Stage I: Involvement of a single lymph node region
Stage II: Involvement of two adjacent lymph node regions on one side of the diaphragm
Stage III: Involvement of lymph node regions on both sides of the diaphragm
Stage IV: Disseminated involvement or an extralymphatic organ with or without associated lymph node involvement

In non-Hodgkin lymphoma the histologic classification is more important than the anatomic dissemination.

Differential Diagnosis

Inflammatory infectious lymphadenopathy	– Small size
	– Associated with infection, inflammatory granulomatous disease (sarcoidosis, Wegener granulomatosis), immune defect, chronic heart failure, etc.
	– Tuberculous lymph nodes—central necrosis, peripheral enhancement
Lymph node metastases	– Usually small size
	– Differential diagnosis is straightforward where there is a known underlying disorder
	– Most common primary tumors include bronchial carcinoma, breast carcinoma, and renal cell carcinoma, melanoma; in carcinoma of unknown primary, these include CUP syndrome, bronchial and breast carcinomas, and germ cell tumors
Castleman disease	– The more common local hyaline vascular type (90% of cases) is characterized by hypervascularity

Selected References

Schiepers C, Filmont JE, Czernin J. PET for staging of Hodgkin's disease and non-Hodgkin's lymphoma. Eur J Nucl Med Mol Imaging 2003; 30: 82–88

Strollo DC, Rosado-de-Christenson ML, Jett JR. Primary mediastinal tumors: Part 2 Tumors of the middle and posterior mediastinum. Chest 1997; 112: 1344–1357

Definition

Benign lymphoproliferative lymph node hyperplasia.

▶ **Epidemiology**

No sex predilection ● Young adults ● HIV patients have a higher risk of multicentric manifestation.

▶ **Etiology, pathophysiology, pathogenesis**

Chronic inflammatory process involving an unknown antigen (multicentric forms are associated with HIV and HHV-8) ● 90% of cases are of the local hyaline vascular type involving follicular lymphocyte proliferation with interfollicular vessels ● 10% are of the plasma cell type, less vascularized, with interfollicular plasma cell bands.

Imaging Signs

▶ **Modality of choice**

CT, MRI.

▶ **Radiographic findings**

Polycyclic mediastinal and/or hilar mass.

▶ **CT findings**

– *Hyaline vascular type:* Lymphomas showing strong homogeneous contrast enhancement (inhomogeneous enhancement results from necrosis, fibrosis, and degeneration); feeding vessels may be present ● Predilection for the middle and posterior mediastinum and central hilar region (anterior mediastinum is rarely involved) ● Calcifications occur in 5–10% of cases.

– *Plasma cell type:* The abdomen and retroperitoneal space are involved in addition to the intrathoracic and extrathoracic regions; cervical involvement is less common ● Slight contrast enhancement.

▶ **MRI findings**

Hyperintense to muscle on T1-weighted sequences ● Hypointense on T2-weighted sequences.

▶ **Pathognomonic findings**

Mediastinal lymphomas showing marked enhancement.

Clinical Aspects

▶ **Typical presentation**

Hyaline vascular type: Asymptomatic, at most with symptoms due to mass effect ● *Plasma cell type:* Fever, fatigue, anemia.

▶ **Confirmation of the diagnosis**

Biopsy.

▶ **Therapeutic options**

Hyaline vascular type: Complete resection or radiation therapy ● *Plasma cell type:* Chemotherapy, antiretroviral therapy, anti-CD20 antibody therapy (rituximab).

Fig. 10.12 Castleman disease in a 30-year-old woman. The plain chest radiograph shows asharply demarcated polycyclic tumor in the right hilum, an asymptomatic incidental finding. The finding is radiographically indistinguishable from other lymphomas or tumors of other etiology. With the hyaline vascular type, the marked enhancement on contrast-enhanced CT can be helpful in identifying the type of lymphoma.

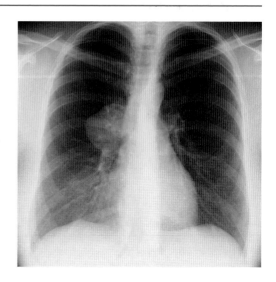

▶ **Course and prognosis**
Hyaline vascular type: Good with complete resection ● *Plasma cell type:* Less favorable.

▶ **What does the clinician want to know?**
Diagnosis and differential diagnosis.

Differential Diagnosis

Lymphoma or leukemia	– Less contrast enhancement
	– Symptomatic
	– Blood count
Neurogenic tumors	– Different location: posterior mediastinum
	– Do not show marked enhancement
Thymic tumors	– Different location: anterior upper mediastinum
	– Do not show marked enhancement
Paragangliomas	– Predilection for the cervical region
Sarcoidosis	– Does not show marked enhancement
	– Pulmonary involvement
Kaposi sarcoma	– HIV
	– Involvement of bronchovascular structures
	– Cutaneous manifestation nearly invariably present

Tips and Pitfalls

Difficulties with differential diagnosis are to be expected especially with the plasma cell variant.

Can be misinterpreted as a malignant lymphoma.

Selected References

Dham A, Peterson BA. Castleman disease. Curr Opin Hematol 2007; 14: 354–359

Hillier JC et al. Imaging features of multicentric Castleman's disease in HIV infection. Clin Radiol 2004; 59: 596–601

Ko SF et al. Imaging spectrum of Castleman's disease. AJR Am J Roentgenol 2004; 182: 769–775

Mediastinal Disorders

Definition

▶ **Epidemiology**
Metastases confined to regional mediastinal lymph nodes are rare.

▶ **Etiology, pathophysiology, pathogenesis**
Most common primary tumors include bronchial carcinoma, breast carcinoma, renal cell carcinoma, and melanoma; in carcinoma of unknown primary, these include bronchial and breast carcinomas and germ cell tumors.

Imaging Signs

▶ **Modality of choice**
CT, MRI, PET/CT.

▶ **CT and MRI findings**
Mediastinal lymph nodes exceeding 10 mm (measured along their short axis) are evaluated as abnormal (subcarinal nodes 15 mm, retrocrural nodes 6 mm) • Hypervascularized metastases (showing contrast enhancement) in renal cell carcinoma, choriocarcinoma, thyroid carcinoma, carcinoid • Lymph node calcifications are inconsistent with a malignancy • Exceptions include metastases of osteochondral tumors, metastases of a mucinous adenocarcinoma, and metastases during or after therapy • Lymph nodes with central necrosis occur in squamous cell carcinoma and tuberculosis.

▶ **PET/CT findings**
Increase in glucose metabolism in malignant processes as well as in acute or chronic inflammatory processes (such as anthracosis) • Only negative findings are of diagnostic value in N staging • Positive findings in tumor staging require histologic examination.

▶ **Pathognomonic findings**
On CT and MRI, size is usually the only criterion of malignancy, albeit an unreliable one • Lymph nodes > 1 cm (measured along the short axis) are classified as abnormal, although the size of mediastinal lymph nodes varies with their location • FDG-PET allows evaluation of malignancy within limits.

Clinical Aspects

▶ **Typical presentation**
Depends on the underlying disorder or initial situation: Asymptomatic incidental finding • Finding in the setting of tumor staging • In the presence of predominant symptoms such as inflow obstruction or dyspnea.

▶ **Therapeutic options**
Depend on the underlying disorder or initial situation • Metastases confined to regional lymph nodes are treated by surgical resection and radiation therapy.

▶ **Course and prognosis**
Depend on the underlying disorder or initial situation • In lung carcinoma 5-year survival is 5–35% • In carcinoma of unknown primary median survival is 3–11 months.

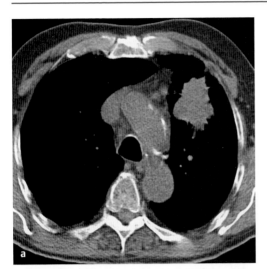

Fig. 10.13 Bronchial carcinoma with mediastinal lymph node metastases (PET/CT). The lymph nodes exhibit borderline size on CT (**a**). PET (**b**) shows increased glucose metabolism indicative of nodal involvement (positive N value).

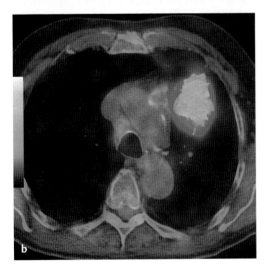

▶ **What does the clinician want to know?**
N staging in the presence of a known tumor ● Where there is no history of tumor, determine whether findings are malignant, perform staging, search for primary tumor.

Differential Diagnosis

Sarcoidosis	– Usually symmetric lymph nodes that are readily distinguishable from each other
Primary malignant lymphoma	– Often massive conglomerate tumors with impairment of the tracheobronchial system and major vessels
	– Small cell lung cancer is an exception
Inflammatory infectious lymphadenopathy	– Pneumonia
	– Tuberculosis
	– Tuberculous lymph nodes more often exhibit central necrosis
	– Clinical and pulmonary findings are crucial to the diagnosis

Tips and Pitfalls

Plain radiographs may show false-negative findings or findings may be misinterpreted as pulmonary arterial hypertension ● Positive CT or MRI findings may be misinterpreted with respect to their malignancy; findings should always be evaluated in their clinical context ● A positive PET finding can be misinterpreted as a malignancy.

Selected References

Dwamena BA et al. Metastases from non-small cell lung cancer: mediastinal staging in the 1990 s-meta-analytic comparison of PET and CT. Radiology 1999; 213: 530–536

Hübner G, Wildfang I, Schmoll HJ. [Metastasen bei unbekanntem Primärtumor—CUP-Syndrom]. In: Schmoll HJ, Höffken K, Possinger K (eds). [Kompendium Internistische Onkologie.] 4 th ed. Heidelberg: Springer; 2006: 5317–5364 [In German]

Riquet M et al. Metastatic thoracic lymph node carcinoma with unknown primary site. Ann Thorac Surg 2003; 75: 244–249

Definition

▶ **Epidemiology**
Ectopic production of blood cells in response to deficient cell production in he-mopoietic bone marrow ● Occurs primarily in the thoracic paravertebral region.

▶ **Etiology, pathophysiology, pathogenesis**
Increased blood production in the setting of a myeloproliferative syndrome (my-elofibrosis, polycythemia) ● Reactive increased erythropoiesis in hemolytic ane-mia (thalassemia, sickle cell anemia) ● Compensatory condition in response to displacement of hemopoietic bone marrow (as in lymphoma or leukemia).

Imaging Signs

▶ **Modality of choice**
MRI.

▶ **Radiographic, CT, and MRI findings**
Paravertebral mass of soft tissue density, typically forming a cuff extending over several segments of the thoracic spine ● CT shows inhomogeneous enhance-ment ● The lesion is of normal intensity to slightly hyperintense on T1-weighted MR images and hyperintense on T2-weighted images ● No bone erosion.

▶ **Nuclear medicine**
Uptake of Tc99 m sulfur colloid.

▶ **Pathognomonic findings**
Paravertebral mass extending over several segments of the thoracic spine.

Clinical Aspects

▶ **Typical presentation**
Usually asymptomatic incidental finding ● Rarely there will be neurologic symp-toms due to spinal cord compression.

▶ **Therapeutic options**
Radiation therapy (neurologic symptoms constitute an emergency) ● Treatment of the underlying disorder.

▶ **Course and prognosis**
Depend on the underlying disorder.

▶ **What does the clinician want to know?**
Spinal cord compression ● Biopsy may be indicated where imaging findings are equivocal ● *Caution:* Risk of hemorrhage.

Fig. 10.14 Extramedullary hemopoiesis in a 47-year-old man with thalassemia.

a The thoracic spine radiograph shows a long spindle-shaped paravertebral shadow extending over several segments.

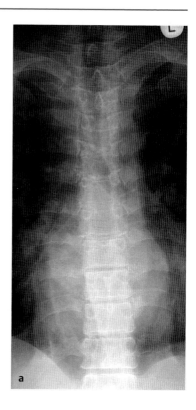

Differential Diagnosis

Neurofibroma or neurilemoma	– Usually unilateral and limited to a few segments – Compressive bone erosion
Paraganglioma	– Usually unilateral – Marked enhancement
Esophageal varices	– Enhancement consistent with blood and vascular structures
Pleural mesothelioma	– Not limited to the paravertebral region
Paravertebral abscess	– Clinical symptoms – Marginal enhancement

Tips and Pitfalls

Can be misinterpreted as a lymphoma. The diagnosis is straightforward in the context of a known underlying disorder.

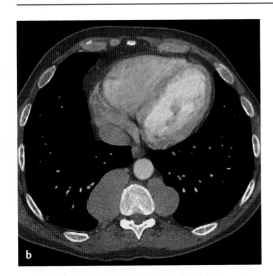

b, c CT visualizes this as a polycyclic, nearly symmetrical mass without bony erosion.

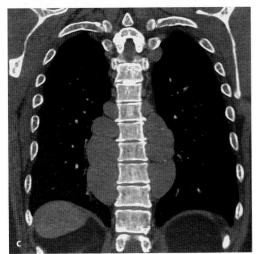

Selected References

Chourmouzi D et al. MRI findings of extramedullary haemopoesis. Eur Radiol 2001; 11: 1803–1806

Gmeinwieser J et al. [Extramedulläre Hämatopoese als Ursache paravertebraler Tumor-bildung im Thorax.] Fortschr Röntgenstr 1982; 137: 68–72 [In German]

Raab BW et al. [Extramedulläre Blutbildung im paravertebralen Raum.] Med Klin 2002; 97: 692–696 [In German]

Definition

▶ **Epidemiology**
A fundamental distinction is made between congenital diaphragmatic hernias (0.04% of live births) and traumatic diaphragmatic hernias (about 1% of cases of blunt trauma, abdominal trauma more often than chest trauma) ● Adult hiatal hernias (> 10% of persons over age 50) represent a distinct entity.

▶ **Etiology, pathophysiology, pathogenesis**
Congenital hernias arise from developmental diaphragmatic defects in typical locations: Bochdalek hernia occurs in the vertebrocostal trigone, accounting for 85–90% of hernias ● Morgagni hernia occurs in the sternocostal triangle (cleft of Larrey), accounting for 1–2% ● Eventration is a hypoplastic diaphragm, accounting for 5%.
Adult hiatal hernia results from weakness of the diaphragmatic musculature around the hiatus ● Age and obesity are predisposing factors.

Imaging Signs

▶ **Modality of choice**
Radiographs, CT.
▶ **Radiographic and CT findings**
– *Hiatal hernia:* Air-containing mass in the left retrocardiac region with or without a fluid level ● Over 90% are axial sliding hiatal hernias (cardia within the chest cavity) ● Less than 5% are paraesophageal hernias (cardia within the abdomen) ● Combined hernia ● The "upside down stomach" is a variant in which more than two-thirds of the stomach herniate into the chest cavity.
– *Bochdalek and Morgagni hernias:* In adults generally appear as a smoothly demarcated mass lying on the diaphragm at a typical posterolateral or anteromedial parasternal location ● They usually contain fatty tissue and therefore appear hypodense.
▶ **Pathognomonic findings**
– *Hiatal hernia:* Air-containing retrocardiac mass with or without a fluid level.
– *Bochdalek and Morgagni hernias:* Circumscribed domelike hump in the diaphragm isodense to fat on CT.

Clinical Aspects

▶ **Typical presentation**
Usually the lesion is an asymptomatic incidental finding ● Rarely, in hiatal hernia symptoms occur, including dysphagia, epigastric pain, gastroesophageal reflux, sensation of pressure and fullness, and occasionally anemia.
▶ **Therapeutic options**
Symptomatic hernia: Surgical correction (hiatal repair, fundoplication).
▶ **Course and prognosis**
Good ● "Upside down stomach" involves a risk of gastric volvulus.

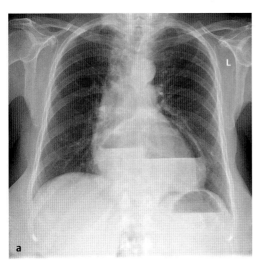

Fig. 10.15 Hiatal hernia in a 65-year-old man. The plain radiographs show—projected on the silhouette of the heart or posterior to it—a broad domelike radiolucency with uniform walls and a double fluid level like an "upside down stomach." A stomach bubble is still visible inferior to the diaphragm.

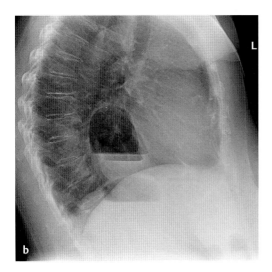

▶ **What does the clinician want to know?**
Identify a hiatal hernia as an axial, paraesophageal, or combined hernia • In a Bochdalek or Morgagni hernia, confirm the tentative diagnosis.

Differential Diagnosis
....

CT can usually provide a straightforward differential diagnosis where radiographic findings are equivocal.

Hiatal hernia	– Esophageal varices—known cirrhosis of the liver with portal hypertension
	– Duplication cyst or bronchogenic cyst
	– Pulmonary sequestration—age of occurrence, systemic arterial supply
Morgagni hernia	– Pleural or pericardial fatty mass
	– Pericardial cyst
Bochdalek hernia	– Neurogenic tumor

Selected References

Eren S, Ciris F. Diaphragmatic hernia: diagnostic approaches with review of the literature. Eur J Radiol 2005; 54: 448–459

Panicek DM et al. The diaphragm: anatomic, pathologic, and radiologic considerations. Radiographics 1988; 8: 385–425

Definition

▶ **Epidemiology**
Circumscribed or continuous dilation of the aorta by more than 50% of its normal diameter (ascending aorta = 4 cm) ● Prevalence is about 4% of the population over age 65 ● Predisposing factors include atherosclerosis, hypertension, trauma ● At-risk individuals include those with connective tissue disorders (Marfan syndrome, Ehlers-Danlos syndrome).

▶ **Etiology, pathophysiology, pathogenesis**
Aneurysm of the ascending aorta due to cystic medial necrosis ● Aneurysm of the descending aorta due to arteriosclerosis ● Lesions are classified according to type (true or false aneurysm), location (ascending or descending aorta), and shape (saccular or fusiform).

Imaging Signs

▶ **Modality of choice**
CTA, MRA.

▶ **Radiographic findings**
Widened, elongated aortic shadow with prominent aortic knob ● Kinking of the descending aorta ● Mural calcifications ● Tracheal shift.

▶ **CTA and MRA**
CT and MRI allow quantitative evaluation and provide information on mural structure, mural thrombi, and possible complications.

▶ **Pathognomonic findings**
Mass along the course of the thoracic aorta ● Widening of the aortic lumen by more than 50%.

Clinical Aspects

▶ **Typical presentation**
Usually the lesion is an asymptomatic incidental finding ● Occasionally there may be dysphagia and hoarseness.

▶ **Therapeutic options**
Management of hypertension.

▶ **Course and prognosis**
Risk of rupture ● Indications for surgery include ascending aortic aneurysm 5.5 cm or larger, descending aortic aneurysm 6.5 cm or larger (smaller in Marfan syndrome), and any symptomatic aneurysm.

▶ **What does the clinician want to know?**
Quantitative evaluation ● Complications and risks.

Fig. 10.16 Asymptomatic saccular thoracic aortic aneurysm in a 43-year-old woman.

a The plain chest radiograph shows a slightly prominent aortic knob with fine mural calcification on the tracheal aspect and a convex protrusion beneath the discoid projection of the aortic arch.

b The trachea and right main bronchus are shifted. The upper mediastinum appears denser on the lateral radiograph. Review of the patient's history revealed previous chest trauma.

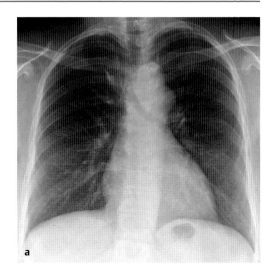

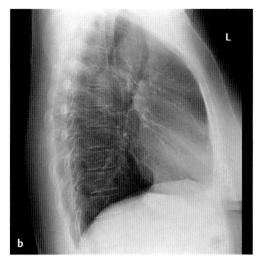

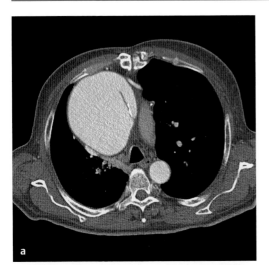

Fig. 10.17 Ascending aortic aneurysm in a 62-year-old man. The CT scans show an extensive aneurysm of the ascending aorta with an intimal flap.

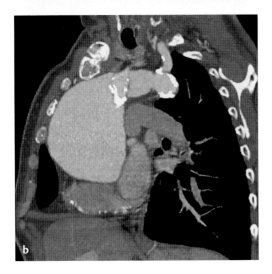

Differential Diagnosis

Poststenotic aortic dilation	– Aortic valve stenosis – Limited to the proximal ascending aorta
Coarctation of the aorta	– Functional narrowing of the descending aorta – Ectasia of the left subclavian artery – Rib notching under certain circumstances
Esophageal achalasia	– Retrotracheal or retrocardiac mass along the esophagus – Air–fluid level

Tips and Pitfalls

Can be misinterpreted as a mediastinal tumor.

Selected References

Posniak HV et al. CT of thoracic aortic aneurysms. Radiographics 1990; 10: 839–855

Definition

Absent or insufficient lower esophageal sphincter relaxation upon swallowing.

▶ **Epidemiology**
Primary achalasia is more common in young people, secondary achalasia in older patients ● No sex predilection.

▶ **Etiology, pathophysiology, pathogenesis**
Primary achalasia involves impaired lower esophageal sphincter relaxation with ganglion cell degeneration in the myenteric plexus of unclear etiology (possibly due to viral infection or an autoimmune process) ● The hypomotile or amotile form is far more common than hypermotile achalasia ● Secondary achalasia occurs where scarring leads to stenosis in reflex esophagitis or secondary to chemical injuries.

Imaging Signs

▶ **Modality of choice**
Barium swallow is preferable to CT.

▶ **Radiographic findings (in hypomotile or amotile form)**
Mediastinal widening with a double contour ● Tubular retrotracheal or retrocardiac mass ● Retrotracheal fluid level ● Gastric air bubble is absent ● Barium swallow shows maximally dilated, fluid-filled esophagus with food ● Contrast medium sedimentation ● Absent or slow peristalsis ● Delayed passage of contrast medium ● Distal esophagus exhibits a "bird beak" deformity.

▶ **CT findings**
Full-length dilation of the esophagus with fluid level, no wall thickening, and abrupt narrowing near the cardia ● No reaction in adjacent tissue or lymphadenopathy.

▶ **Pathognomonic findings**
Maximally dilated, distally narrowed esophagus with slow peristalsis and delayed passage of contrast medium into the stomach.

Clinical Aspects

▶ **Typical presentation**
Dysphagia ● Recurrent aspiration pneumonia.

▶ **Therapeutic options**
Pneumatic dilation ● Myotomy.

▶ **What does the clinician want to know?**
Diagnosis ● Severity of functional impairment.

Fig. 10.19 Esophageal achalasia. The plain chest radiograph shows a mediastinal shadow abnormally widened on the right side without a cardiac silhouette sign. The right paracardiac projection of the mass exhibits an air–fluid level at the level of the hilum, which is suggestive of esophageal achalasia (not a cranially displaced stomach).

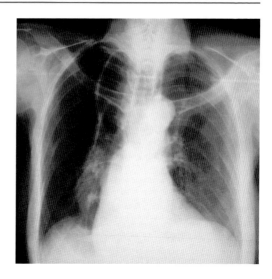

Differential Diagnosis

Achalasia secondary to carcinoma of the gastroesophageal junction	– Irregular tumorous thickening of the wall and narrowing of the lumen – Only moderate prestenotic dilatation – Lymphadenopathy – Rapid development – Cachexia
Scarring with esophageal stenosis	– History – Gastroesophageal reflux – Distal stenosis with at most only moderate dilatation – Chemical injury – Changes over a longer distance – Impaired motility – Variable prestenotic dilatation of the lumen
Chagas disease	– Enlarged esophagus due to destruction of intramural ganglion cells (endemic in South America; caused by *Trypanosoma cruzi*) – Other organ manifestations

Tips and Pitfalls

Can be mistaken for mediastinal lymphadenopathy.

Selected Reference

Hannig C, Wuttge-Hannig A, Rummeny E. [Motilitätsstörungen des Ösophagus.] Radiologe 2007; 47: 123–136 [In German]

Definition

▶ **Epidemiology**
Incidence is 6 : 10 000 per year ● Three times as common in men than in women ●
Generally occurs in advanced age (> 60) ● Predisposing factors include hypertension, Marfan syndrome, and Ehlers–Danlos syndrome.

▶ **Etiology, pathophysiology, pathogenesis**
Cystic intimal necrosis leads to an intimal tear with subintimal hematoma which progresses to mural dissection ● *Stanford classification:* A type A dissection involves the ascending aorta; a type B dissection begins distal to the origin of the left subclavian artery ● A chronic dissection is a dissection older than 2 weeks.

Imaging Signs

▶ **Modality of choice**
CTA, MRA.

▶ **Radiographic findings**
Widening of the upper mediastinum ● Double contour of the aortic knob ● Intimal calcification separated from the aortic wall (> 1 cm) ● Rupture is accompanied by an "apical cap," pleural effusion, and/or pericardial effusion ● Findings are negative in 25 % of cases.

▶ **CTA, MRA findings**
Helical intraluminal intimal flap ● The false lumen lies in a right anterolateral position in the ascending aorta and in a left posterolateral position in the descending aorta ● The false lumen may show significantly delayed contrast filling.

▶ **Pathognomonic findings**
Intimal flap demonstrated.

Clinical Aspects

▶ **Typical presentation**
Chest pain radiating into the back ● Weak pulse ● Shock ● Neurologic deficits occur in about 20 % of cases ● Signs of ischemia due to deficient perfusion of organs and extremities ● Clinically silent dissection occurs in 10 %, especially in Marfan syndrome.

▶ **Therapeutic options**
Type A dissection is treated surgically ● Type B dissection is treated conservatively by reducing blood pressure; dissected aneurysms > 5 cm are treated surgically.

▶ **Course and prognosis**
High mortality if left untreated.

▶ **What does the clinician want to know?**
Type of dissection ● Complications (rupture, impaired perfusion).

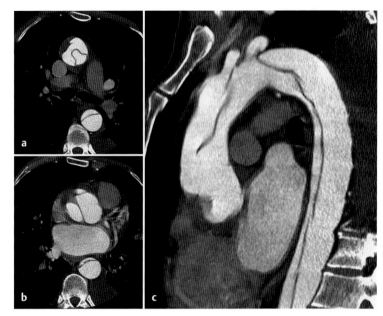

Fig. 10.20 Axial (**a**, **b**) and sagittal oblique (**c**) CT-images of a type A dissection in a 57-year-old man. A long intimal flap beginning in the ascending aorta and continuing into the descending aorta and involving the supraaortic branches.

Differential Diagnosis

Aortic aneurysm	– An aneurysm with a mural thrombus can be difficult to distinguish from a dissection with a completely thrombosed false lumen
Mediastinal tumor	– Differential diagnosis is straightforward on cross-sectional imaging studies

Tips and Pitfalls

A streak artifact (straight line with variable orientation) can mimic a dissection •
Delayed contrast filling of the false lumen can mimic thrombosis (obtain a second delayed series).

Selected References

Theisen D et al. CT angiography of the aorta. Radiologe 2007; 47: 982–992
Willoteaux S et al. Imaging of aortic dissection by helical CT. Eur Radiol 2004; 14: 1999–2008

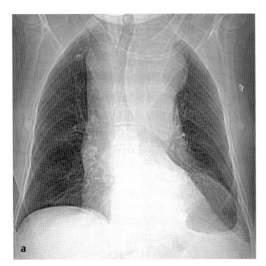

Fig. 10.21 Dissection in aortic ectasia with kinking in an 85-year-old man.

a The plain chest radiograph shows a massive widening of the upper mediastinum with prominent aortic knob.

b CTA demonstrates a type B dissection (relatively narrow false lumen) with signs of rupture and an extensive mediastinal hematoma.

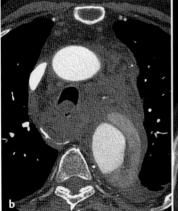
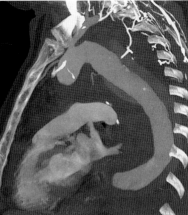

Definition

Membranous stenosis of the thoracic aorta at the isthmus distal to the origin of the left subclavian artery.

▶ **Epidemiology**

Occurs in about 5 : 1000 births ● Accounts for 5–10% of congenital defects ● Twice as common in men than in women ● Associated with Turner syndrome, bicuspid aortic valve, and ventricular septal defect.

▶ **Etiology, pathophysiology, pathogenesis**

Developmental anomaly ● Collateral circulation via the intercostal arteries and mammary branches.

Imaging Signs

▶ **Modality of choice**

Ultrasound in children, MRA or CTA in adults and for follow-up.

▶ **Radiographic findings**

Slender aortic knob with double convexity (superior contour is the left subclavian artery, inferior contour is the poststenotic dilation of the aortic arch) ● inverse ε sign ● Rib notching is not invariably present and is not visible before age 6.

▶ **MRA, CTA**

These modalities directly visualize the coarctation ● MRI can quantify the stenosis by flow measurement and estimation of the pressure gradients.

▶ **Pathognomonic findings**

Direct visualization of the coarctation.

Clinical Aspects

▶ **Typical presentation**

Often an asymptomatic incidental finding in the diagnostic workup of hypertension ● Difference in blood pressure between the upper and lower extremities.

▶ **Therapeutic options**

Surgical or interventional correction.

▶ **Course and prognosis**

Prognosis is good with adequate correction ● Follow-up is indicated.

▶ **What does the clinician want to know?**

Hemodynamic significance ● Quantification ● Associated malformations.

Differential Diagnosis

Pseudocoarctation	– Congenital elongation of the aorta with kinking at the level of the ligamentum arteriosum
	– High-riding elongated aorta without stenosis
Rib notching	– Pseudoerosion in neurofibromatosis (twisted ribs)
	– Collaterals in obstruction of the pulmonary artery

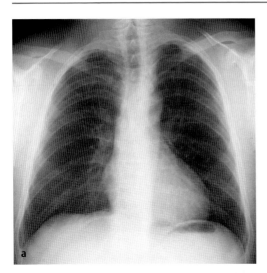

Fig. 10.22 Coarctation of the aorta in a 54-year-old woman.

a The plain chest radiograph. The heart appears more prominent on the left and there is a faint double contour of the aortic knob, with a cranial extension forming a shadow band (the expanded left subclavian artery). Bilateral rib notching.

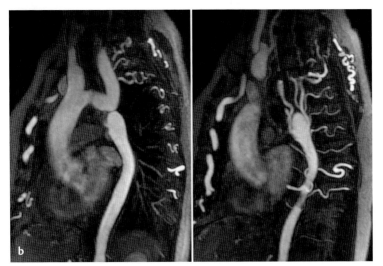

b The MR image shows a high-grade coarctation of the aorta with well-developed collaterals via the intercostal and mammary arteries. Functionally expanded left subclavian artery.

Mediastinal Disorders

Tips and Pitfalls

Failure to adequately investigate associated malformations.

Selected References

Kinsara A, Chan KL. Noninvasive imaging modalities in coarctation of the aorta. Chest 2004; 126: 1016–1018

Nielsen JC et al. MRI predictors of coarctation severity. Circulation 2005; 111: 622–628

Definition

▶ **Epidemiology**
Anomalies of the aortic arch occur in about 1% of the population • No sex predilection.

▶ **Etiology, pathophysiology, pathogenesis**
Defective obliteration of the symmetric branchial arterial arches and dorsal aorta; several variants exist.
– *Right aortic arch* with aberrant origin of the left subclavian artery arising as the last vessel from the aortic arch after the left carotid, right carotid, and right subclavian arteries • Most common form • Usually occurs without an associated heart defect (10% of cases) • Asymptomatic.
– *Right aortic arch* with mirror-image origin of the supra-aortic branches (left subclavian, left carotid, right carotid, and right subclavian arteries) • Often associated with heart defects (90% of cases).
– *Duplication of the aortic arch:* The carotid artery or subclavian artery arises from the arch of the same name • The arches merge posterior to the esophagus into the descending aorta along the midline • Usually there is a dominant right arch and a left descending aorta (75% of cases).

Imaging Signs

▶ **Modality of choice**
CTA, MRA.

▶ **Radiographic findings**
– *Right aortic arch:* No aortic knob on the left • Aortic knob appears in a right paratracheal position, impressing the trachea and displacing it to the left.
– *Duplication of the aortic arch:* Aortic knobs appear on both sides of the trachea and esophagus • The trachea courses along the midline and is impressed by the dominant arch (the right aortic arch is usually larger and higher than the left one) • The descending aorta courses along the midline • The trachea and esophagus are shifted anteriorly at the level of the aortic arch.

▶ **CTA, MRA**
These modalities definitively delineate the anomalous vascular anatomy and associated findings • In duplication of the aortic arch, axial images demonstrate how both aortic arches arise from the ascending aorta, enclose the trachea and esophagus, and give rise to one carotid and one subclavian artery each.

▶ **Pathognomonic findings**
See "Radiographic findings."

Clinical Aspects

▶ **Typical presentation**
Right aortic arch with aberrant origin of the left subclavian artery, usually asymptomatic • Symptomatic anomalies with stridor, recurrent infections, and dysphagia from tracheal and esophageal compression include duplication of the aortic

Fig. 10.23 The plain chest radiograph shows a right aortic arch in a 25-year-old man. There is no aortic knob on the left. Instead it appears in a right paratracheal position (atypically high) displacing the trachea slightly to the left. Right descending aorta.

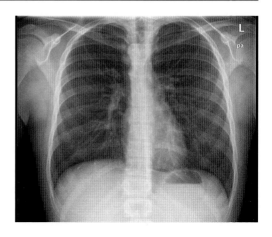

arch, right descending aorta with left ductus arteriosus, and arteria lusoria • Symptoms usually occur in early childhood.

▶ **Therapeutic options**
Asymptomatic anomalies require no treatment, in other cases surgical correction.

▶ **Course and prognosis**
Depend on any associated heart defects.

▶ **What does the clinician want to know?**
Classification • Determine the cause • Preoperative planning if necessary.

Differential Diagnosis

Mediastinal tumor	– Differential diagnosis is straightforward on cross-sectional imaging studies
Aberrant left pulmonary artery, pulmonary sling	– Atypical course of the left pulmonary artery between the trachea and esophagus: posterior impression of the trachea, anterior impression of the esophagus

Tips and Pitfalls

A right aortic arch with a left descending aorta coursing leftward posterior to the trachea suggests duplication of the aortic arch with an atretic left segment • A right aortic arch in which the aberrant left subclavian artery arises from an aortic diverticulum (of Kommerell) can mimic duplication of the aortic arch or a tumor.

Selected References

Jaffe RB. Radiographic manifestations of congenital anomalies of the aortic arch. Radiol Clin North Am 1991; 29: 319–334

Steiner RM et al. Congenital heart disease in the adult patient: The value of plain film chest radiology. J Thorac Imaging 1995; 10: 1–25

Mediastinal Disorders

Definition

Widening of the azygos vein to over 10 mm when standing and 15 mm in the supine position.

▶ **Etiology, pathophysiology, pathogenesis**
Congenital aplasia of the suprarenal vena cava produces a primary anomaly with an "azygos continuation" of the inferior vena cava ● Dilation may also occur in collateral circulation secondary to obstruction or obliteration of the inferior vena cava or terminal segment of the superior vena cava (rare).

Imaging Signs

▶ **Modality of choice**
CT, MRI (CTA, MRA).
▶ **Radiographic findings**
Significantly widened and rounded azygos vein shadow.
▶ **CT and MRI findings**
Functionally expanded azygos and hemiazygos veins in congenital aplasia of the suprarenal vena cava (azygos continuation of the inferior vena cava) or obstruction of the vena cava.
▶ **Pathognomonic findings**
A finding of azygos dilatation is pathognomonic, given the unequivocal anatomic situation.

Clinical Aspects

▶ **Typical presentation**
Usually asymptomatic incidental finding.
▶ **Therapeutic options**
Depend on the cause and/or finding.
▶ **Course and prognosis**
Depend on the cause and/or finding.
▶ **What does the clinician want to know?**
Determine the cause and exclude a tumor.

Differential Diagnosis

Right aortic arch or duplication of the aortic arch	– Right tracheal shift and/or impression – Normal venous anatomy
Superior vena cava syndrome	– Distal occlusion of the superior vena cava by a tumor with a normal inferior vena cava
Hypervolemia	– Normal venous anatomy – Signs of increased pulmonary perfusion
Lymphadenopathy	– Normal venous anatomy

Fig. 10.24 Dilated azygos vein and extensive venous thromboses in a 48-year-old woman with recurrent thromboses in a coagulation disorder with AT-III, protein C, and protein S deficiency.

a The plain chest radiograph shows significant dilatation of the azygos vein shadow in the angle between the trachea and right main bronchus. The trachea and main bronchus are neither shifted nor impressed. Pleural effusion on the left side.

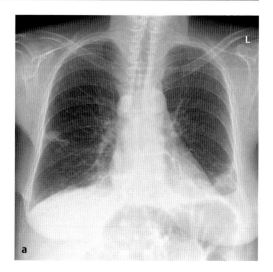

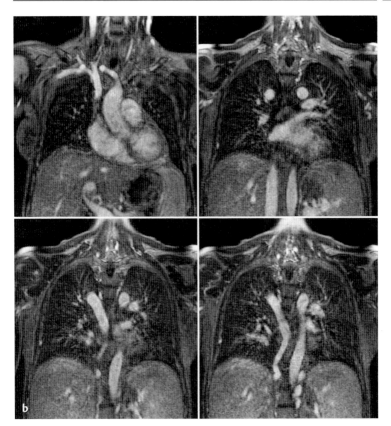

b The MR images show occlusion of the superior vena cava caudal to the junction of the azygos vein. Venous drainage of the upper half of the body occurs with retrograde perfusion via the azygos system.

Tips and Pitfalls

An incidental finding without clinical significance can be misinterpreted as relevant pathology.

Selected References

Schaefer-Prokop C. Mediastinum, pleura and chest wall. In: Galanski M, Prokop M (eds.). Computed Tomography of the Body. Stuttgart: Thieme; 2003: 373–404

Yilmaz E et al. Interruption of the inferior vena cava with azygos/hemiazygos continuation accompanied by distinct renal vein anomalies: MRA and CT assessment. Abdom Imaging 2003; 28: 392–394

Definition

▶ **Epidemiology**
The mediastinal space communicates cranially with the cervical soft tissue and caudally with the abdomen. This means that inflammatory processes can spread by direct extension into the mediastinum.

▶ **Etiology, pathophysiology, pathogenesis**
Acute mediastinitis occurs secondary to traumatic or iatrogenic esophageal perforation or spontaneous rupture (Boerhaave syndrome) in 90% of cases ● Spread of infection from the cervical region or abdomen (pancreatitis) ● Sequela of thoracic surgery.
Fibrosing mediastinitis can occur due to: Specific infection ● Radiation therapy ● Methysergide therapy ● As an idiopathic disorder ● Often associated with other fibrosing disorders.

Imaging Signs

▶ **Modality of choice**
MRI is preferable to CT ● Barium swallow is indicated in any suspected esophageal perforation.

▶ **Radiographic findings**
Findings are negative or unspecific (blurred contours, widened mediastinal shadow).

▶ **CT and MRI findings**
  – *Acute mediastinitis:* Diffusely increased density with pronounced mediastinal fatty tissue and obliteration of mediastinal structures ● Hyperintense on T2-weighted sequences ● Intraluminal administration of contrast medium is indicated to identify the perforation.
  – *Fibrosing mediastinitis:* Localized or generalized, can also occur as a mass obstructing the vena cava, tracheobronchial system, and pulmonary vessels ● Intermediate signal intensity on T1-weighted sequences, heterogeneously hyperintense and hypointense on T2-weighted sequences ● Calcifications occur in the localized form in 60–80% of cases.

▶ **Pathognomonic findings**
  – *Acute mediastinitis:* History and clinical findings are crucial to the diagnosis.
  – *Fibrosing mediastinitis:* Signs of obstruction of the vena cava, tracheobronchial system, and/or pulmonary vessels in the generalized form ● Calcifications in the localized form.

Clinical Aspects

▶ **Typical presentation**
  – *Acute mediastinitis:* Chest pain ● Fever ● Sepsis.
  – *Fibrosing mediastinitis:* Asymptomatic or with signs of obstruction of the vena cava, pulmonary veins, trachea, or esophagus.

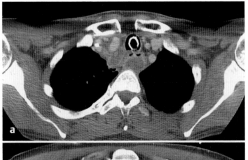

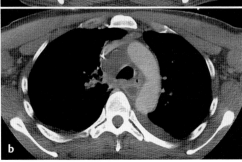

Fig. 10.25 Mediastinal abscess in a 44-year-old man. The contrast CT scans demonstrate liquid formations paratracheal and paraesophageal with significant marginal enhancement of uniform width marking the abscess membrane. These findings originated from a descending parapharyngeal abscess.

▶ **Therapeutic options**
  – *Acute mediastinitis:* Antibiotics • Drainage • Revision surgery.
  – *Fibrosing mediastinitis:* Steroids • Surgery • Local intervention.
▶ **Course and prognosis**
  – *Acute mediastinitis:* High mortality if left untreated.
  – *Fibrosing mediastinitis:* Long protracted history, airway compromise, or respiratory failure.
▶ **What does the clinician want to know?**
  Abscess • Location and extent • Is intervention indicated?

Differential Diagnosis

Fibrosing mediastinitis	– Lymphoma—circumscribed mass, hyperintense on T2-weighted sequences
	– Erdheim–Chester disease: Diaphyseal and metaphyseal bone changes (cortical thickening, medullary sclerosis)

Tips and Pitfalls

Depending on the findings, there is a risk of overstating or understating their clinical significance.

Selected References

Rossi SE et al. Fibrosing mediastinitis. Radiographics 2001; 21: 737–757

Definition

▶ **Epidemiology**
  Most common thoracic deformity.
▶ **Etiology, pathophysiology, pathogenesis**
  Developmental anomaly, usually clinically silent ▪ Often associated with mitral valve prolapse.

Imaging Signs

▶ **Modality of choice**
  Radiographs, CT.
▶ **Radiographic findings**
  Right paramediastinal opacity with slight leftward shift of the heart shadow so that the right margin of the heart is no longer concurrent with the right margin of the mediastinum ▪ On the lateral film, the sternum appears significantly posterior to the anterior contour of the ribs ▪ The retrocardiac space is significantly narrowed.
▶ **CT findings**
  The axial image shows marked indentation of the sternum with loss of the normal convexity of the anterior chest wall, which instead appears concave.
▶ **Pathognomonic findings**
  See the radiographic and CT findings.

Clinical Aspects

▶ **Typical presentation**
  Usually an asymptomatic incidental finding.
▶ **Therapeutic options**
  Surgical correction is indicated where the ratio between the transverse and sagittal thoracic axes ("pectus index") is greater than 3.25.
▶ **What does the clinician want to know?**
  Severity and whether surgery is indicated.

Differential Diagnosis

Middle-lobe atelectasis	– Normal sternum
Middle-lobe pneumonia	– Clinical aspects
	– Normal sternum

Tips and Pitfalls

Can be misinterpreted as middle lobe pathology.

Selected Reference

Goretsky MJ et al. Chest wall abnormalities: pectus excavatum and pectus carinatum. Adolec Med Clin 2004; 15: 455–471

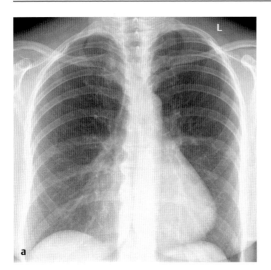

Fig. 11.1 Pectus excavatum in a 60-year-old woman. The plain chest radiograph (**a**) shows an opacity in the right paramediastinal lower lung field with a slight leftward shift of the heart silhouette. The contour of the heart is not concurrent with the right margin of the mediastinum. The findings suggest pectus excavatum. The lateral film (**b**) confirms this diagnosis.

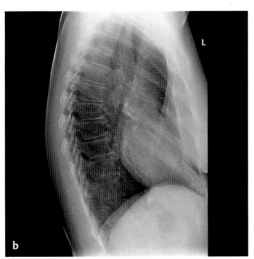

Definition

Air in the pleural space.

▶ **Epidemiology**
Most often a sequela of trauma or biopsy ● Spontaneous pneumothorax has an annual incidence of 10 : 10 000.

▶ **Etiology, pathophysiology, pathogenesis**
Primary: Spontaneous pneumothorax ● Often associated with apical bullae and hereditary connective tissue disorders (Marfan syndrome, Ehlers–Danlos syndrome).
Secondary: Traumatic ● Iatrogenic ● Emphysema ● Sarcoidosis ● Cystic lung disease (lymphangioleiomyomatosis, Langerhans cell histiocytosis) ● Parainfectious or postinfectious (*Pneumocystis jirovecii* pneumonia, staphylococcal pneumonia) ● Neoplastic (metastases of osteosarcoma).

Imaging Signs

▶ **Modality of choice**
Plain chest radiograph (expiration film is not required).

▶ **Radiographic findings**
Pleural line parallel to the chest wall with a space free of pulmonary parenchyma lateral to the lung itself ● *Note:* Typical signs can be absent in chest radiographs obtained in the supine patient ● Signs of anterior pneumothorax include a deep sulcus, unusually sharp diaphragmatic, cardiac, and mediastinal contours and increased transradiancy in the upper abdomen ● Tension pneumothorax is characterized by mediastinal shift and a flattened, caudally shifted diaphragmatic dome.

▶ **CT findings**
Directly visualizes the air-filled pleural space ● Even anterior pneumothorax is readily demonstrated.

▶ **Pathognomonic findings**
Pleural line with a space free of pulmonary parenchyma.

Clinical Aspects

▶ **Typical presentation**
Sudden chest pain (90% of cases) and dyspnea (80%).

▶ **Therapeutic options**
Drainage ● Bullectomy or pleurodesis may be indicated to treat recurrent pneumothorax ● Tension pneumothorax and recurrent pneumothorax require treatment ● Treatment is advisable in pneumothorax exceeding 25% of the volume of the hemithorax or about 500 mL.

▶ **Course and prognosis**
Usually good.

▶ **What does the clinician want to know?**
Demonstrate lesion ● Extent.

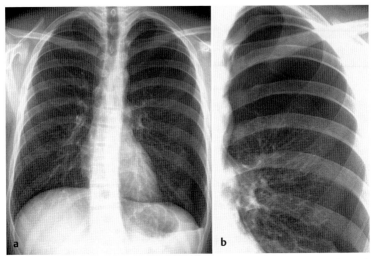

Fig. 11.2 Spontaneous pneumothorax in a 17-year-old boy. The plain chest radiograph shows a mantle of avascular space around the left lung, bordered by a medial pleural line. The paramediastinal portion of the lung creates an unusually sharp contour of the aortic knob.

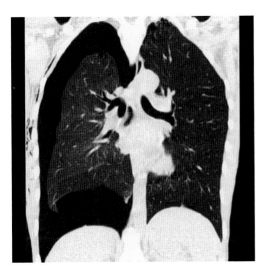

Fig. 11.3 Tension pneumothorax in a 27-year-old man. CT shows severe, mantlelike pneumothorax in the right lung with midline shift to the left and a flattened and displaced right diaphragmatic dome.

Differential Diagnosis

Bullous emphysema	– CT is recommended to differentiate this from encapsulated pneumothorax
Artifact, skin or drape fold	– Mach effect (either stopping short of or entering the pleural space) that mimics a pleural line

Tips and Pitfalls

False-negative or -positive findings.

Selected References

Seow A et al. Comparison of upright inspiratory and expiratory chest radiographs for detecting pneumothoraces. AJR Am J Roentgenol 1997; 166: 313

Wintermark M, Duvoisin B, Schnyder P. Trauma of the pleura. In: Schnyder P, Wintermark M (eds.). Radiology of blunt trauma of the chest. Berlin, Heidelberg, New York: Springer; 2000: 57–70

Definition

▶ **Epidemiology**
Common causes include increased hydrostatic pressure (heart failure), reduced plasma osmotic pressure (in cirrhosis of the liver, nephrotic syndrome, renal insufficiency), infection, pneumonia • Less common causes include tumors, transdiaphragmatic passage of ascites, and collagen diseases.

▶ **Etiology, pathophysiology, pathogenesis**
Transudate: Increased hydrostatic capillary pressure or reduced plasma osmotic pressure, protein concentration of 1.5–2.5g/dL • *Exudate:* Increased capillary permeability (inflammatory or neoplastic), protein concentration > 3g/dL, lactate dehydrogenase > 200 IU, protein concentration ratio of pleural fluid to serum > 0.5, lactate dehydrogenase in pleural fluid ≥ 2/3 of serum lactate dehydrogenase.

Imaging Signs

▶ **Modality of choice**
Ultrasound, plain chest radiographs.

▶ **Ultrasound findings**
Anechoic or hypoechoic band posterior to the chest wall demarcated by hyperechoic visceral pleura, which contrasts against the lung • Echo inhomogeneities, septa, and pleural thickening suggest an exudate.

▶ **Radiographic findings**
Findings depend on the extent of the effusion and patient position (erect or supine) • With increased volume of effusion there is rounding of the costophrenic angles • Lateralization of the diaphragmatic dome in subpulmonary effusion, distance between the gastric air bubble and base of the lung > 1.5 cm • Obliteration of the diaphragmatic contour and loss of retrodiaphragmatic vascularity • Basal shadow with meniscus sign • Hemithorax shadow with mediastinal shift • *With the patient supine:* Reduced transparency of the hemithorax and apical cap.

▶ **CT findings**
Effusion initially accumulates in the posterior pleural recess • Several signs distinguish pleural effusion from abdominal fluid—diaphragm sign (pleural fluid lies outside the diaphragmatic contour) • Interface sign (fluid is sharply demarcated from liver or spleen in ascites) • Displaced crus sign (pleural effusion displaces the diaphragmatic crus cranially and anteriorly) • Bare area sign (ascites separates the liver from the diaphragm only as far as the coronary ligaments).

▶ **Pathognomonic findings**
See "Radiographic findings."

Fig. 11.4 Massive pleural effusion on the right side in a 60-year-old man. The plain chest radiograph shows a full, homogeneously dense shadow in the right lower half of the chest. The lateral portion of the shadow rises like a meniscus, extending here to the minor interlobar fissure.

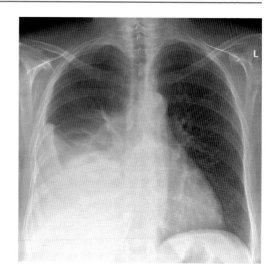

Clinical Aspects

▶ **Typical presentation**
Dyspnea depending on the volume of effusion and the underlying disorder.

▶ **Therapeutic options**
Depend on the underlying disorder.

▶ **Course and prognosis**
Depend on the underlying disorder.

▶ **What does the clinician want to know?**
Etiology ● Drainage of encapsulated fluid accumulations.

Differential Diagnosis

Malignant pleural effusion	– Often massive – Unilateral – Nodular pleural thickening in pleural metastases – Positive cytology
Tuberculous pleural effusion	– Protein-rich (75g/dL) – High lymphocyte content (> 70%) – Positive culture in only 25% of cases
Empyema	– Enhancement of visceral and parietal pleura – Split pleura sign
Collagen diseases	– Especially systemic lupus erythematosus, Wegener granulomatosis, rheumatoid arthritis
Chylothorax	– Density is 0 HU or less – Most common cause is trauma or lymphoma

Tips and Pitfalls

Difficulty distinguishing pleural effusion from infradiaphragmatic intraabdominal fluid accumulations (see "CT findings").

Selected References

Müller NL. Imaging of the pleura. Radiology 1993; 186: 297–309

Raasch BN et al. Pleural effusion: Explanation of some typical appearances. AJR Am J Roentgenol 1982; 139: 899–904

Definition

▶ **Epidemiology**
Occurs in: Pleural effusion • Pleural empyema • Hemothorax • Chylothorax • Pneumoconiosis • Pleuropulmonary infections.

▶ **Etiology, pathophysiology, pathogenesis**
Localized or extensive scarred adhesions of both pleural membranes, occasionally with calcifications.

Imaging Signs

▶ **Modality of choice**
CT is preferable to plain radiography.

▶ **Radiographic and CT findings**
Smoothly contoured area densities in the pleura with variable morphology, location, and size • *For example:* Basal from a pleural effusion • Apical from tuberculous pleuropneumonia (simultaneous induration of the upper lobe) • Bilateral with calcific plaques in asbestos exposure • Fibrothorax from hemothorax.

▶ **Pathognomonic findings**
Pleural thickening independent of posture and constant over time.

Clinical Aspects

▶ **Typical presentation**
Usually the lesion is an asymptomatic incidental finding • Dyspnea on exercise may occur where lesions restrict respiratory excursion.

▶ **Therapeutic options**
Decortication in symptomatic cases where lesions restrict respiratory excursion.

▶ **Course and prognosis**
Usually the course is uncomplicated with a good prognosis • Rarely there are complications due to shrinkage of the lesions and scarring with emphysema • In severe cases there may be consequent chest deformities such as scoliosis.

Differential Diagnosis

Pleural effusion	– Temporary finding that varies with posture
	– Lesser density
	– No calcifications
Pleural malignancy	– Nodular pleural changes
	– Contrast enhancement
	– Extrapulmonary focal lesion or pathology
	– History

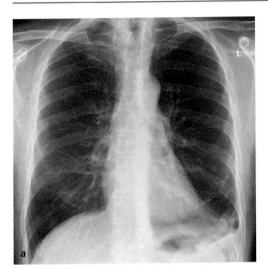

Fig. 11.5 Pleural peel. Left laterobasal pleural fibrosis secondary to pleuropneumonia: **a** plain chest radiograph; and **b** CT.

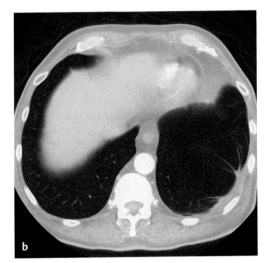

Tips and Pitfalls

A single radiograph without a thorough history will not always be sufficient to distinguish this from a pleural effusion • Ultrasound may be indicated.

Selected References

Müller NL. Imaging of the pleura. Radiology 1993; 186: 297–309

Definition

▶ **Etiology, pathophysiology, pathogenesis**
Usually a sequela of pleuropneumonia or pulmonary abscess • Less often a sequela of thoracic surgery, trauma, or direct extension of another disease process (osteomyelitis in a rib, subphrenic abscess).

Imaging Signs

▶ **Modality of choice**
CT is preferable to plain radiography.
▶ **Radiographic findings**
Extrapleural mass that merges with the chest wall.
▶ **CT findings**
Crescentic or lentiform extrapulmonary mass at an oblique angle to the chest wall • Sharply demarcated from the lung • Compression of adjacent pulmonary parenchyma • Uniform marginal enhancement with more or less smooth interior contour • Split pleura sign • Thickening of the extrapleural subcostal soft tissue.
▶ **Pathognomonic findings**
See "CT findings" • Especially split pleura sign.

Clinical Aspects

▶ **Typical presentation**
Chest pain • General signs of infection.
▶ **Therapeutic options**
Drainage • Surgical removal with decortication where indicated.
▶ **Course and prognosis**
With proper treatment, the prognosis is good.
▶ **What does the clinician want to know?**
Differentiate empyema from abscess • Efficiency of drainage or other therapy.

Differential Diagnosis

Pulmonary abscess	– More spherical
	– Irregular wall with ill-defined junction with pulmonary parenchyma
	– Abrupt termination of bronchovascular structures
	– No compression
Encapsulated pleural effusion	– At most linear marginal enhancement
	– Homogeneous water-equivalent density on CT
	– History of heart failure

Tips and Pitfalls

The radiographic morphology of chronic pleural fluid accumulations can neither confirm nor exclude the presence of superinfection.

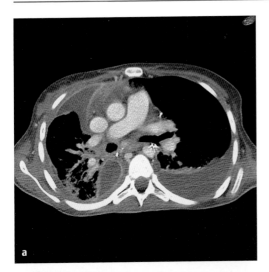

Fig. 11.6 Pleural empyema in an 18-year-old woman with staphylococcal infection following lung transplantation. The cross-sectional images show encapsulated fluid accumulations on the right side (some crescentic and some oval in shape), exhibiting pronounced, uniform marginal enhancement consistent with empyema. An accumulation of free fluid without marginal enhancement is seen in the left posterobasal region. This finding is consistent with a bland pleural effusion.

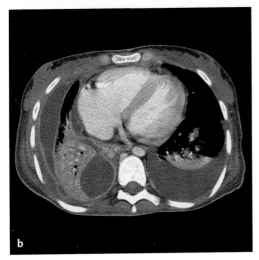

Selected References

Evans AL, Gleeson FV. Radiology in pleural disease: state of the art. Respirology 2004; 9: 300–312

Müller NL. Imaging of the pleura. Radiology 1993; 186: 297–309

Definition

▶ **Epidemiology**
Occupational disease (inhalation of asbestos fibers used in the production of in-
sulation, etc.) • Manifests itself 20–40 years after the start of chronic exposure.

▶ **Etiology, pathophysiology, pathogenesis**
Asbestos-associated changes—asbestos fibers (20–150 µm) penetrate the visceral
pleura, causing small hematomas that later calcify.

Imaging Signs

▶ **Modality of choice**
CT.

▶ **Radiographic findings**
Partially calcified pleural thickening occurring primarily in the subcostal and diaphragmatic regions • Recurrent pleural effusion.

▶ **CT findings**
Plateaulike pleural plaques with or without calcifications in a typical location (see
"Radiographic findings").

▶ **Pathognomonic findings**
Calcified pleural plaques in a typical location with a history of occupational exposure.

Clinical Aspects

▶ **Typical presentation**
Initially there is often an asymptomatic effusion • Symptoms often occur only
20 years after exposure • Symptoms are often caused by pulmonary changes or
a tumor.

▶ **Course and prognosis**
Malignancies: Risk of bronchial carcinoma is 50 times higher in smokers with
chronic exposure • Pleural mesothelioma • Extrathoracic carcinomas (gastrointestinal tract, larynx, etc.).

▶ **What does the clinician want to know?**
International Labour Organization classification • Tumor.

Differential Diagnosis

Postinfectious or posttraumatic pleural thickening	– Calluses are shaped differently and occur at other locations – History

Tips and Pitfalls

The diagnosis is straightforward when a patient with a known history of occupational exposure exhibits typical pathology.

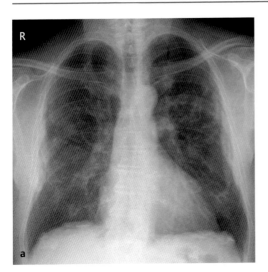

Fig. 11.7 Pleural plaques in a 68-year-old man.

a The plain chest radiograph shows bilateral nodular to patchy pleural calcifications, in part associated with areas of pleural thickening.

b CT visualizes these lesions as plateaulike pleural plaques with the calcifications following the contour of the ribs.

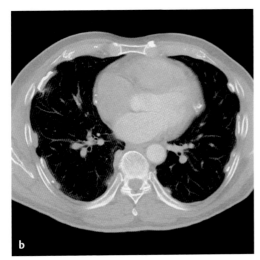

Selected References

Cugell DW, Kamp DW. Asbestosis and the pleura: A review. Chest 2004; 125: 1103–1117

Kim K et al. Imaging of occupational lung disease. Radiographics 2001; 21: 1371–1391

Definition

▶ **Epidemiology**
Mixed infection with aerobic and anaerobic bacteria, usually *Actinomyces israelii* (a normal constituent of oral flora) ● Poor dental hygiene ● *Locations:* Craniofacial region (55%), abdominal and pelvic region (20%), thoracic region (15%), mixed (10%).

▶ **Etiology, pathophysiology, pathogenesis**
A. israelii enters deeper layers through a break in the mucosa or via aspiration into the lung ● This leads to bronchopulmonary infections and infiltration of the pleura and chest wall ● A cervical fascial infection can also spread to the chest by direct extension.

Imaging Signs

▶ **Modality of choice**
CT.

▶ **Radiographic findings**
Nonsegmental infiltrate (usually in the peripheral upper lobe) with involvement of the pleura and chest wall.

▶ **CT findings**
Infiltrate that disregards fissures and fascial boundaries and spreads within the mediastinum, pleura, and chest wall ● Leads to abscess formation, cavitation, and pleural empyema, and causes costal osteomyelitis with periosteal apposition ● Mediastinal and hilar lymphadenopathy.

▶ **Pathognomonic findings**
Infection that does not respect compartmental boundaries ● Chronic infection with involvement of the pleura and chest wall (empyema, periostitis).

Clinical Aspects

▶ **Typical presentation**
Patients with predilection for aspiration (alcoholics, etc.) ● Cough (initially nonproductive) ● Hemoptysis ● Subfebrile temperature ● Weight loss ● Malaise ● Localized chest pain ● Symptoms of pleuritis.

▶ **Therapeutic options**
High-dose penicillin ● Surgery: Resection of necrotic areas ● Pleural decortication.

▶ **Course and prognosis**
Chronic pneumonia, associated with pleuritis, abscess formation, and fibrosis ● Fistulas ● With early diagnosis and proper treatment, the prognosis is good ● Chronic infection may lead to hypertrophic osteoarthropathy and in some cases secondary amyloidosis.

▶ **What does the clinician want to know?**
Abscess formation ● Chest wall infiltration if present ● Is surgical treatment indicated?

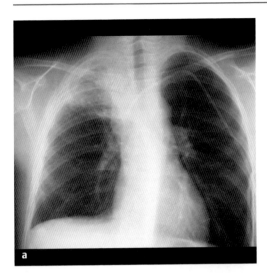

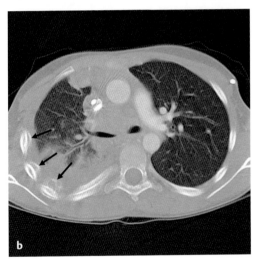

Fig. 11.8 Actinomycosis in a 10-year-old boy with a history of nonproductive cough over several months, who had been referred to an orthopedist for postural deformity and rubbery swelling above the scapula. The plain chest radiograph (**a**) and CT (**b**) show extensive infiltration of the right upper lobe with associated pleural soft tissue band and widening of the upper mediastinum without tracheal shift or constriction. On CT (**b**) the area of consolidation appears homogeneously dense with a partial air bronchogram. The right hemithorax is slightly flattened. The key finding is the presence of broad areas of periosteal apposition without associated bony destruction.

Differential Diagnosis

Empyema necessitatis *Penetrating empyema*	– Other mycotic infections that tend to spread to the chest wall (aspergillosis, blastomycosis, crypto-coccosis, nocardiosis) – Tuberculosis
Pneumonia *(bacterial or mycotic)*	– Isolated pathogen – Course
Bronchial carcinoma	– History of smoking – Age

Tips and Pitfalls

Clinical and radiologic pictures in the acute phase are nonspecific • The disorder can mimic bronchial carcinoma as it does not respect anatomic boundaries (biopsy is often indicated).

Selected References

Conant EF, Wechsler RJ. Actinomycosis and nocardiosis of the lung. J Thorac Imaging 1992; 7: 75–84

Kim TS et al. Thoracic actinomycosis: CT features with histopathologic correlation. AJR Am J Roentgenol 2006; 186: 225–231

Mabeza GF, Macfarlane J. Pulmonary actinomycosis. Eur Respir J 2003; 21: 545–551

Definition

▶ **Epidemiology**
Of all pleural tumors, 95% are metastases ● Primary malignant pleural tumors are much more common than benign ones.

▶ **Etiology, pathophysiology, pathogenesis**
In 80% of cases, pleural mesothelioma occurs secondary to asbestos exposure after a mean latency period of 35 years ● It is usually epithelial, less often sarcomatous or mixed.

Imaging Signs

▶ **Modality of choice**
CT.

▶ **Radiographic findings**
Irregular nodular, focal, or multifocal pleural thickening without any mediastinal shift.

▶ **CT findings**
Identical to radiographic findings ● Involvement of the interlobar pleura occurs in 80% of all cases, pleural effusion in 75%, volume loss in the affected hemithorax in 40% ● Extrapleural infiltration (lung, pericardium, chest wall, ribs) is a criterion of malignancy ● Pleural thickening, nodular lesions, circular lesions, mediastinal lesions, interlobar pleural involvement, rapidly recurring pleural effusion, and abnormal lymph nodes (tracheobronchial, hilar, parasternal, diaphragmatic) are suggestive of malignancy.

▶ **MRI findings**
The lesion appears isointense to slightly hyperintense on T1-weighted sequences, and slightly hyperintense on T2-weighted sequences ● More sensitive in detecting infiltration (chest wall, mediastinum, diaphragm).

▶ **PET**
Suitable for N staging.

▶ **Pathognomonic findings**
Irregular nodular tumorous pleural thickening without any mediastinal shift but with involvement of the interlobar pleura and recurrent pleural effusion.

Clinical Aspects

▶ **Typical presentation**
Intense unilateral chest pain ● Cough ● Dyspnea ● Recurrent pleural effusion.

▶ **Confirmation of the diagnosis**
Pleural biopsy.

▶ **Therapeutic options**
Criteria for resectability include: No extrapleural tumor infiltration ● No contralateral lymph node metastases ● No distant metastases.

Fig. 11.9 Pleural meso-thelioma in a 78-year-old man. In the right hemi-thorax, which on the whole is reduced in size, the plain chest radio-graph (**a**) and CT scan (**b**) show coarse nodular pleural tumors affecting all segments of the pleura, including the mediastinal and dia-phragmatic areas. Asso-ciated posterobasal pleural effusion is also present.

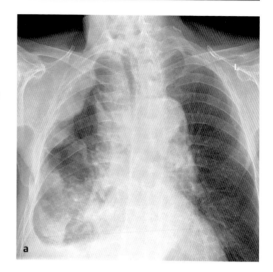

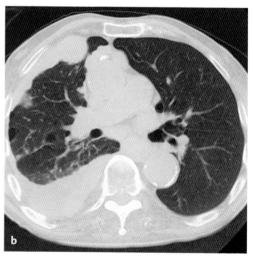

▶ **Course and prognosis**
  Prognosis is not favorable • 5–year survival is less than 25%.
▶ **What does the clinician want to know?**
  Evaluation of malignancy • Staging.

Differential Diagnosis

Pleural metastases	– Bronchial carcinoma (40%), breast carcinoma (25%), thymic carcinoma
Hemangioendothelioma	– Rare – Similar growth pattern but less pleural thickening
Endometriosis	– Nodular pleural thickening with pain that varies with the menstrual cycle and hemothorax
Intrathoracic splenosis	– History of trauma with rupture of the spleen and diaphragm
Encapsulated pleural effusion	– History of heart failure – Formation of pleural fibrin bodies
Pleural empyema	– History of pneumonia (usually posterobasal) and split pleura sign
Benign pleural tumors	– No signs of infiltration – Heterogeneous appearance that can include cystic, hemorrhagic, and necrotic components – Radiographically indistinguishable

Tips and Pitfalls

Degree of infiltration is often underestimated on CT.

Selected Reference

Benamore RE, O' Doherty MJ, Entwisle JJ. Use of imaging in the management of malignant pleural mesothelioma. Clin Radiol 2005; 60: 1237–1247

Definition

▶ **Epidemiology**
Most common pleural tumors • Benign pleural tumors (lipoma, fibroma) are very rare.

▶ **Etiology, pathophysiology, pathogenesis**
Usually these are metastases of adenocarcinomas (40% of bronchial carcinomas, 20% breast carcinomas, less often carcinomas of the gastrointestinal tract or female sex organs) or lymphomas • The pathogenetic mechanism involves hematogenous or lymphatic spread, or direct invasion.

Imaging Signs

▶ **Modality of choice**
CT.

▶ **Radiographic findings**
Pleural effusion is usually the first, and often the only, sign.

▶ **CT findings**
Pleural effusion is seen in combination with usually multilocular nodular, less often uniform pleural thickening and increased contrast enhancement • Areas of nodular pleural thickening, extensive circular pleural thickening, involvement of the mediastinal pleura, and areas of parietal pleural thickening measuring more than 1 cm are suggestive of malignancy.

▶ **Pathognomonic findings**
Disseminated areas of pleural thickening • Severe pleural effusion refractory to treatment.

Clinical Aspects

▶ **Typical presentation**
Dyspnea with increasing effusion.

▶ **Therapeutic options**
Treatment of the underlying disorder • Pleurodesis in symptomatic effusion.

▶ **Course and prognosis**
This depends on the type and stage of the malignant tumor.

Differential Diagnosis

Pleural mesothelioma	– Usually radiographically indistinguishable from pleural metastases
	– Usually unilateral and asbestos-associated (latency period up to 40 years)
	– Pleural plaques

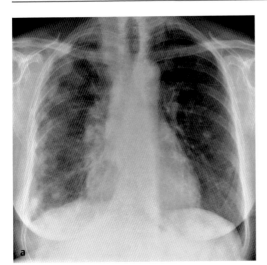

Fig. 11.10 Pleural metastases in a 65-year-old woman with thyroid carcinoma. The plain chest radiograph (**a**) and CT (**b**) show multiple pleural tumor nodules on the right side, forming a mantle that encloses the lung, including the mediastinal pleura. Only isolated nodules are seen on the left side.

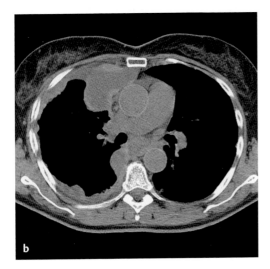

Pleural empyema or fibrothorax	– Encapsulated pleural effusion in the acute stage, occasionally with air inclusions
	– Split pleura sign
	– History and clinical findings
Splenosis	– Asymptomatic
	– History of multiple trauma with rupture of the spleen and diaphragm
Invasive thymoma	– Pleural invasion without pleural effusion
Solitary pleural tumors	– Asymptomatic incidental findings of variable size
	– Usually benign
	– Lipoma: fat-equivalent density
	– Fibroma is sessile or pedunculated, usually arises from the visceral pleura, and shows inhomogeneous enhancement

Tips and Pitfalls

Experience has shown that areas of pleural thickening suggestive of malignancy are usually visible only after drainage of the effusion.

Selected References

Dynes MC et al. Imaging manifestations of pleural tumors. Radiographics 1992; 12: 1191–1201

Leung AN, Müller NL, Miller RR. CT in differential diagnosis of diffuse pleural disease. AJR Am J Roentgenol 1990; 154: 487–492

Müller NL. Imaging of the pleura. Radiology 1993; 186: 297–309

Definition

▶ **Epidemiology**
Pulmonary contusions and lacerations represent different degrees of damage to the pulmonary parenchyma; these injuries account for 30–60% of all chest trauma • Main causes in everyday life include: Motor vehicle accidents (about 75% of cases) • Falls from a great height (18%) • Occupational accidents (7%) • Rarely, stab or gunshot wounds (depending on local environmental factors).

▶ **Etiology, pathophysiology, pathogenesis**
A distinction is made between blunt and penetrating chest trauma, depending on the mechanism of injury • Acceleration/deceleration forces predominate in severe chest trauma • Variants include blast injuries, which involve a shock wave • Shock wave trauma leads to severe tears along the air–tissue interfaces • There is a risk of air embolism, and prompt artificial respiration is required.

Imaging Signs

▶ **Modality of choice**
Radiographs • CT in severe chest trauma and multiple trauma.

▶ **Radiographic findings**
Homogeneous opacity with an ill-defined border • Laceration is distinguishable from contusion only by the presence of pneumatoceles or dense hematoma • Findings manifest themselves within hours of the injury • Contusions resolve within days; lacerations heal in weeks to months.

▶ **CT findings**
A contusion appears as an ill-defined minimally invasive area of increased density resembling a ground-glass opacity • Lacerations are denser and more inhomogeneous • Air inclusions with air–fluid levels are consistent with traumatic pneumatoceles.

Clinical Aspects

▶ **Typical presentation**
Pulmonary contusions and lacerations are usually clinically asymptomatic • Gas exchange is impaired only where there is extensive parenchymal damage with associated injuries (unstable chest, pneumothorax, hemothorax) • Blast injuries are invariably associated with respiratory insufficiency.

▶ **What does the clinician want to know?**
Extent of injury • Associated injuries requiring treatment (hemothorax, pneumothorax, tension pneumothorax, unstable chest, aortic rupture, rupture of the diaphragm).

Fig. 12.1 Multiple trauma in a 16-year-old boy.
a The plain chest radiograph shows coarsely nodular to patchy densities over both lungs.
b The CT scan allows better differentiation between the contused areas (arrows), and the lacerations with pneumatoceles (open arrows).

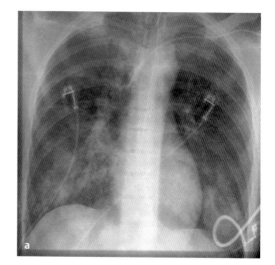

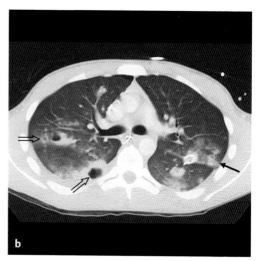

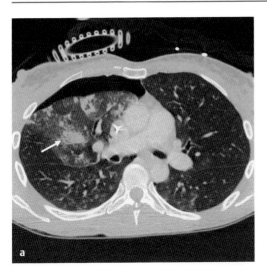

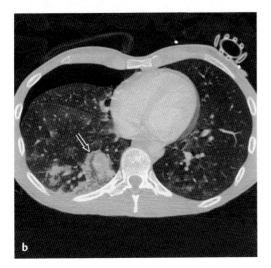

Fig. 12.2 Multiple trauma. The CT scans show a right anterior pneumothorax. Contused areas appear as ill-defined areas of nodular opacification (arrow), and hematomas from lacerations as denser sharply demarcated focal lesions (open arrow).

Chest Trauma

Differential Diagnosis

Sequelae of aspiration	– Gravitational location and segmental distribution
	– Sequelae of trauma do not respect anatomic borders except for the interlobar fissures
Atelectasis	– Volume loss of varying degrees
	– Uniform enhancement on contrast CT

Tips and Pitfalls

In contrast to CT, less extensive associated pleural injuries (pneumothorax or hemothorax) are easily overlooked on plain chest radiographs • Such injuries usually do not require treatment.

Selected Reference

Schnyder P, Wintermark M. Radiology of blunt trauma of the chest. Berlin: Springer; 2000

Definition

▶ **Epidemiology**
Aortic ruptures occur in about 1–2% of all cases of chest trauma (> 80% are fatal) ●
Traffic accidents are the most common cause.

▶ **Etiology, pathophysiology, pathogenesis**
Acceleration/deceleration forces predominate in severe chest trauma ● Injury
typically occurs at the aortic isthmus (descending aorta distal to the origin of the
subclavian artery).

Imaging Signs

▶ **Modality of choice**
CTA.

▶ **Radiographic findings**
Abnormal widening of the upper mediastinum (> 8 cm) in combination with
signs of a mass (trachea and esophagus shifted to the right; left main bronchus is
also shifted) ● High negative predictive value where plain chest radiograph is normal (98%).

▶ **CTA findings**
Aortic rupture on CTA appears as an abrupt change in caliber ● Abnormal aortic
contour ● Intimal flap ● Intramural and/or periaortic hematoma.

Clinical Aspects

▶ **Typical presentation**
Cardinal symptom of aortic rupture is shock, a sign of which may be a difference
in blood pressure between the right and left arms or between the upper and lower halves of the body.

▶ **What does the clinician want to know?**
Confirm and localize or exclude ● Hemothorax ● Associated injuries.

Differential Diagnosis

Mediastinal hematoma	– Most mediastinal hematomas are caused by bleeding from smaller vessels
	– Wherever mediastinal widening is observed in the setting of trauma, one must consider the possibility of a spinal fracture in addition to vascular injury

Tips and Pitfalls

Pulsation artifacts can mimic aortic dissection (pulsation artifacts change direction
and location in every slice).

Chest Trauma

Fig. 12.3 Contained aortic rupture in a 40-year-old man with multiple trauma.

a The plain chest radiograph shows widening of the upper mediastinum. The knob of the aorta is no longer clearly distinguishable although the contour descending aorta still is. The left main bronchus is elongated and displaced. There is slight tracheal shift.

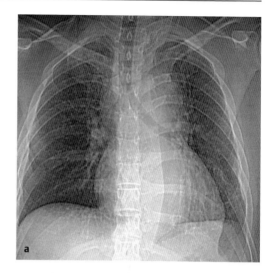

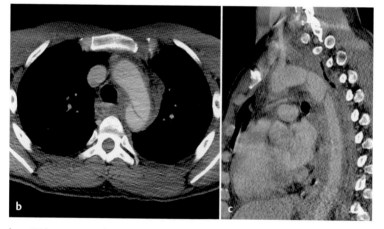

b, c CT demonstrates the aortic rupture at a typical location distal to the origin of the subclavian artery, with an intimal flap. There is an associated periaortic hematoma.

Selected Reference

Wintermark M, Wicky S, Schnyder P. Imaging of acute traumatic injuries of the thoracic aorta. Eur Radiol 2002; 12: 432–442

Definition

▶ **Epidemiology**
Accounts for less than 1% of all cases of chest trauma.
▶ **Etiology, pathophysiology, pathogenesis**
Invariably occurs in the setting of severe chest trauma • Acceleration/deceleration forces predominate • Injuries typically occur in the main bronchus, near the carina.

Imaging Signs

▶ **Modality of choice**
CT.
▶ **Radiographic findings**
Signs include pneumothorax or pneumomediastinum refractory to treatment • Atelectasis refractory to treatment.
▶ **CT findings**
Interruption or step-off in the contour or discontinuity of the course of the main bronchus • "Fallen lung" sign (the right upper lobe bronchus with its anterior segmental bronchus no longer lies at the level of the carina but farther caudal and now exhibits an oblique posterior course).

Clinical Aspects

▶ **Typical presentation**
Tracheobronchial ruptures are usually missed initially.
▶ **What does the clinician want to know?**
Confirm and localize the injury.

Differential Diagnosis

Mediastinal emphysema – Barotrauma due to artificial respiration

Tips and Pitfalls

The injury can be overlooked because with few exceptions there are no direct signs • Bronchoscopy is indicated where such an injury is suspected.

Selected References

Wintermark M et al. Trauma of the mediastinum. In: Schnyder P, Wintermark M (eds). Radiology of blunt trauma of the chest. Berlin: Springer; 2000

Fig. 12.4 Bronchial rupture in a 36-year-old woman involved in a motor vehicle accident. The coronal CT image (slab) shows mediastinal emphysema. The right main bronchus appears discontinuous. There is no evidence of collapse of the right lung or tension pneumothorax.

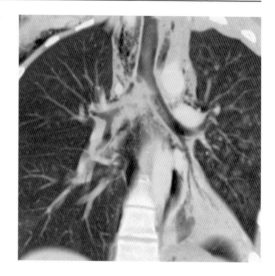

Definition

▶ **Epidemiology**
Esophageal rupture due to endoscopy (60% of esophageal ruptures), forced vomiting (15%), and chest trauma (10%).

▶ **Etiology, pathophysiology, pathogenesis**
Penetrating trauma, usually iatrogenic (endoscopy, surgery), causes most ruptures. The cause less often is increased intraluminal pressure or Boerhaave syndrome and least often it is thoracic trauma ● The posterolateral wall of the distal esophagus is the weakest point, with a thin muscular layer and little soft tissue coverage.

Imaging Signs

▶ **Modality of choice**
CT with oral contrast administration in applicable cases, Barium swallow.

▶ **Radiographic findings**
Pneumomediastinum ● Subcutaneous emphysema ● Pleural effusion or hydropneumothorax (on the left in rupture of the distal esophagus, on the right in rupture of the middle or proximal esophagus) ● Contrast extravasation on Barium swallow (false-negative findings in about 20% of cases).

▶ **CT findings**
Paraesophageal air and fluid accumulations ● Otherwise identical to radiographic findings ● Iatrogenic injury commonly occurs where the lumen is physiologically or pathologically narrowed; blunt chest trauma and Boerhaave syndrome usually rupture the distal esophagus.

▶ **Pathognomonic findings**
Contrast extravasation after oral administration.

Clinical Aspects

▶ **Typical presentation**
Deep chest pain ● Dysphagia ● Hematemesis ● Subcutaneous emphysema ● History.

▶ **Confirmation of the diagnosis**
Endoscopy ● Contrast extravasation on CT Barium swallow.

▶ **Therapeutic options**
Surgical repair and drainage ● Antibiotics.

▶ **Course and prognosis**
Prognosis depends on the time elapsed between rupture and treatment. Mortality can be as high as 50%.

▶ **What does the clinician want to know?**
Identify and localize ● Complications.

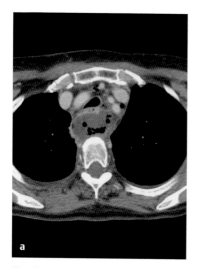 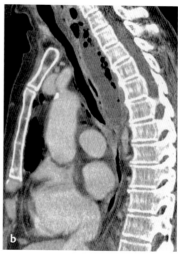

Fig. 12.5 Iatrogenic esophageal perforation in a 76-year-old man. The CT scans show extended fluid accumulation with mass effect and air inclusions posterior to the trachea and esophagus.

Differential Diagnosis

Hiatal or paraesophageal hernia	– History – No pneumomediastinum – No contrast extravasation
Esophageal fistula	– Due to tumor – History

Tips and Pitfalls

A delay in diagnostic examinations may be disadvantageous ● An esophageal rupture should be considered wherever history and clinical findings suggest that possibility.

Selected References

Fadoo FD et al. Helical CT esophagography for the evaluation of suspected esophageal perforation or rupture. AJR Am J Roentgenol 2004; 182: 1177–1179

Gimenez A et al. Thoracic complications of esophageal disorders. Radiographics 2002; 22: 247–258

Definition

▶ **Epidemiology**
Ruptures of the diaphragm are more common in blunt abdominal trauma (3–5% of all cases) than in blunt chest trauma (about 1%).

▶ **Etiology, pathophysiology, pathogenesis**
Three-quarters of ruptures of the diaphragm occur on the left side.

Imaging Signs

▶ **Modality of choice**
CT.

▶ **Radiographs**
Herniation of the abdominal organs into the chest cavity ● Mediastinal shift.

▶ **CT**
Herniation of abdominal organs into the chest cavity ● The contour of the diaphragm is interrupted or missing (sagittal and coronal multiplanar reconstructions are crucial) ● *Dependent viscera sign:* Because of the ruptured diaphragm, the upper abdominal organs are no longer held in their typical positions but recede posteriorly and are in contact with the posterior chest wall over a broad area.

Clinical Aspects

▶ **Typical presentation**
Associated injuries usually dominate the clinical picture, masking the diaphragmatic injury.

▶ **What does the clinician want to know?**
Confirm and localize the rupture ● Herniated organs ● Associated injuries.

Differential Diagnosis

Relaxation of the diaphragm	– Double diaphragmatic dome, elevated anteriorly, more often on the right side
Phrenic palsy	– Contour of the diaphragm remains intact – Deep narrow costophrenic angles – Normal position of abdominal organs
Pulmonary laceration with pneumatoceles	– Contour of the diaphragm remains intact
Congenital diaphragmatic hernia	– Diaphragmatic defect occurs in typical location – Posterior Bochdalek hernia – Parasternal Morgagni hernia

Fig. 12.6 Rupture of the left diaphragm in a 54-year-old woman. The coronal image shows the gastric fundus and parts of the colon that have herniated into the chest cavity. Broad, traumatic diaphragmatic defect with a spurlike lateral diaphragmatic stump (arrow).

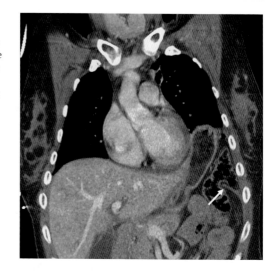

Fig. 12.7 Rupture of the right diaphragm in a 56-year-old man. The plain chest radiograph shows a shadow in the lower half of the right hemithorax with isolated fluid levels and air inclusions. Considered in conjunction with the known abdominal trauma, the findings suggest a rupture of the diaphragm.

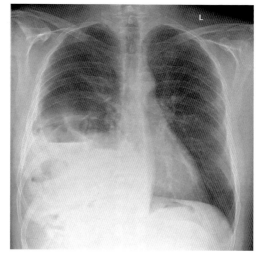

Tips and Pitfalls

Assisted ventilation can mask a rupture of the diaphragm (herniation of the abdominal organs is suppressed).

Selected References

Bergin D et al. The dependant viscera sign in CT diagnosis of blunt traumatic diaphragmatic rupture. AJR Am J Roentgenol 2001; 177: 1137–1140

Shackletom KL, Stewart ET, Taylor AJ. Traumatic diaphragmatic injuries: spectrum of radiographic findings. Radiographics 1998; 18: 49–59

Definition

▶ **Epidemiology**
Lung damage with severe acute respiratory distress.

▶ **Etiology, pathophysiology, pathogenesis**
Causes are chest trauma, fat embolism, sepsis, inhalation of toxic gases, burns, shock, metabolic derangement, drug reactions, etc. • The disorder progresses in several pathoanatomic stages with alveolar capillary damage and formation of hyaline membranes:
  - *Early exudative phase (hours):* Endothelial and interstitial edema.
  - *Late exudative phase (days):* Progressive interstitial/alveolar edema with hemorrhage and alveolar necrosis.
  - *Proliferative phase (weeks):* Exudate organization • Proliferation of alveolar cells and fibroblasts.
  - *Late phase (months):* Repair • Fibrosis.

Imaging Signs

▶ **Modality of choice**
Radiographs • Indications for CT include complications, quantitative estimation, and residual findings.

▶ **Radiographic findings**
For the initial 12–24 hours (latency period) imaging findings are normal despite severe clinical symptoms (dyspnea) • Findings after 24 hours include progressive and increasingly confluent bilateral, primarily peripheral nodular opacities and an air bronchogram • Later findings under artificial respiration with positive end-expiratory pressure (PEEP) include increased transradiancy of the lung fields (a "cosmetic" effect that mimics improvement) and occasionally barotrauma (pneumomediastinum, pneumothorax, interstitial emphysema) • Later, these changes give way to fibrosis and the lung fields show increased transradiancy.

▶ **CT findings**
This modality is more sensitive in detecting early changes, complications, and barotrauma • Often there is a mixed picture of ground-glass and acinar opacities • Usually there is an anteroposterior gradient (hypostasis; depending on the cause) • Residual fibrotic changes typically show a reversed posteroanterior gradient due to protection of the posterior atelectatic parenchymal segments against PEEP oxygen respiration.

▶ **Pathognomonic findings**
Bilaterally symmetric, confluent opacities with or without an air bronchogram • Imaging findings should be interpreted in the context of the clinical picture.

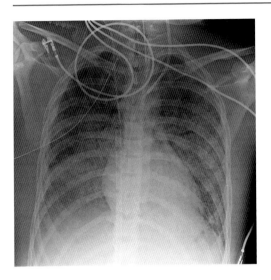

Fig. 12.8 Adult respiratory distress syndrome in a 19-year-old man. He had progressive respiratory insufficiency of uncertain etiology with pulmonary hemorrhages, and the outcome was fatal. The plain chest radiograph shows massive opacification of both lungs with residual ventilated portions only in the upper lung fields.

Clinical Aspects

▶ **Typical presentation**
Acute onset with dyspnea and hypoxemia despite administration of oxygen.
▶ **Therapeutic options**
Artificial respiration ● Infection prophylaxis ● Supportive treatment.
▶ **Course and prognosis**
Mortality is about 40%, usually due to multiple organ failure.
▶ **What does the clinician want to know?**
Complications (especially pneumonia) ● Follow-up.

Differential Diagnosis

Atelectasis or pneumonia	– Differential diagnosis is difficult
	– Progressive focal consolidations and cavitations suggest pneumonia (differential diagnosis should consider pneumatoceles under PEEP respiration)
Atypical pneumonia (Pneumocystis or viral pneumonia)	– Predisposing underlying disease
	– Exposure
	– Febrile clinical syndrome
	– *Pneumocystis jirovecii* pneumonia produces a more uniform, primarily interstitial picture

Acute interstitial pneumonia	– Identical clinical findings and radiographic morphology – Idiopathic – No history of a causative or predisposing disorder
Hydrostatic pulmonary edema	– Underlying cardiac disease – Pleural effusion

Tips and Pitfalls

The diagnosis is usually straightforward in the context of the history and clinical findings • Differentiating pneumonic infiltrates (superinfection) requires clinical data as radiographic findings alone are equivocal.

Selected References

Caironi P, Carlesso E, Gattioni L. Radiological imaging in acute lung injury and acute respiratory distress syndrome. Semin Respir Crit Care Med 2006; 27: 404–415

Goodman LR et al. Adult respiratory distress syndrome due to pulmonary and extrapulmonary causes: CT, clinical, and functional correlations. Radiology 1999; 213: 545

Ware LB, Matthay MA. The acute respiratory distress syndrome. N Engl J Med 2000; 342: 1334–1349

Definition

▶ **Epidemiology**
Occurs primarily with chemotherapy agents (in up to 10% of cases), antiarrhythmic agents (amiodarone), and antiseptic agents (nitrofurantoin), etc.
▶ **Etiology, pathophysiology, pathogenesis**
Purely toxic or immunologic reaction with variable, unspecific manifestation:
Diffuse alveolar damage • Unspecific pneumonitis • Bronchiolitis obliterans with organizing pneumonia • Eosinophilic pneumonia.

Imaging Signs

▶ **Modality of choice**
CT is preferable to plain radiography.
▶ **Radiographic and CT findings**
  - *Diffuse alveolar damage:* Bilateral ground-glass opacification that may include consolidations • Especially busulfan.
  - *Nonspecific interstitial pneumonitis:* Disseminated nodular ground-glass opacities and consolidations in addition to reticular changes, predominantly basal • Especially amiodarone, methotrexate, and carmustine.
  - *Bronchiolitis obliterans with organizing pneumonia:* Nodular ground-glass opacities and consolidations, predominantly peripheral • Especially bleomycin, methotrexate, cyclophosphamide, amiodarone, nitrofurantoin, etc.
  - *Eosinophilic pneumonia:* Nodular ground-glass opacities and consolidations, predominantly in the peripheral upper lobes • Especially nitrofurantoin, penicillamine, antiinflammatory agents, and paraaminosalicylic acid.
▶ **Pathognomonic findings**
Nonspecific findings • Occurrence of symptoms concurrently with therapy is an important diagnostic criterion.

Clinical Aspects

▶ **Typical presentation**
Nonspecific symptoms such as fever, malaise, nonproductive cough, and dyspnea of variable severity • Restrictive ventilation defect.
▶ **Therapeutic options**
Alternative treatment.
▶ **Course and prognosis**
Variable.
▶ **What does the clinician want to know?**
Tentative diagnosis in conjunction with a suggestive constellation of findings.

Fig. 13.1 Sirolimus reaction in a 71-year-old man receiving immunosuppressant macrolide therapy after kidney transplantation. CT shows predominantly basal ground-glass opacities with predominantly interstitial structures similar to findings in nonspecific interstitial pneumonitis.

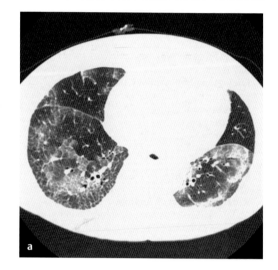

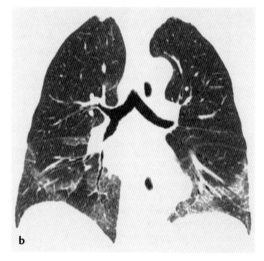

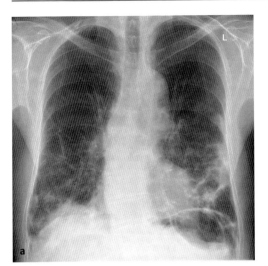

Fig. 13.2 Pulmonary nitrofurantoin reaction in a 73-year-old man. Both the plain chest radiograph (**a**) and CT (**b**) show predominantly basal and peripheral nodular consolidations along with streaky densities similar to findings in bronchiolitis obliterans with organizing pneumonia.

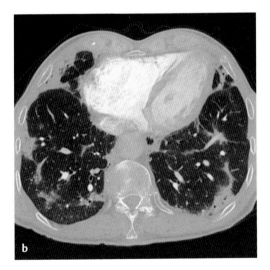

Fig. 13.3 Pulmonary amiodarone reaction in a 70-year-old man.

a The plain chest radiograph shows heterogeneous interstitial shadowing (mixed pattern of streaky reticular shadows and ground-glass confluent opacities) in the right middle and upper lung fields and in the left upper lung field.

b CT also shows a mixed picture—most closely resembling nonspecific interstitial pneumonitis. Areas of normal parenchyma alternate with affected areas. Slight bilateral pleural effusion.

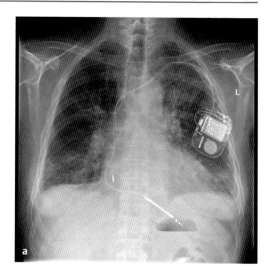

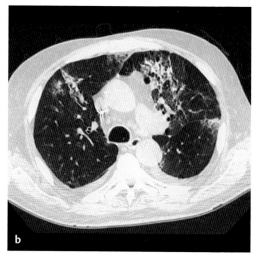

Differential Diagnosis

Pneumonic infiltrates	– Morphologically indistinguishable
	– Clinical findings are crucial to the diagnosis
	– Biopsy may be indicated
Pneumonitis, radiation reaction	– Limited to the irradiated field
Various forms of idiopathic interstitial pneumonia	– Morphologically indistinguishable
	– An initial clinical situation with no history of medication is crucial to the diagnosis

Tips and Pitfalls

Pulmonary changes can be misinterpreted as attributable to causes other than medication, especially when they do not occur concurrently with therapy.

Selected References

Erasmus JJ, McAdams HP, Rossi SE. Drug-induced lung injury. Seminars Roentgenol 2002; 37: 72–81

Erasmus JJ, McAdams HP, Rossi SE. High-resolution CT of drug-induced lung disease. Radiol Clin North Am 2002; 40: 61–72

Definition

▶ **Epidemiology**
Affects 5–10% of patients receiving radiation therapy in the chest • Depends on the irradiated volume, radiation dose and fractionation, and concurrent chemotherapy • Rarely occurs at doses < 30 Gy, nearly invariably at doses > 40 Gy.

▶ **Etiology, pathophysiology, pathogenesis**
Early reaction consists of radiation pneumonitis 1–3 months after therapy and diffuse alveolar damage with an intraalveolar exudate and formation of hyaline membranes • Late reaction consists of radiation fibrosis 6–12 months after therapy or complete recovery.

Imaging Signs

▶ **Modality of choice**
CT is preferable to plain radiography.

▶ **Radiographic and CT findings**
Changes are essentially limited to the irradiated volume • Early reaction consists of a ground-glass opacity or consolidation • Late reaction occasionally consists of fibrosis with signs of volume loss and development of traction bronchiectasis.

▶ **Pathognomonic findings**
Changes not correlating with specific anatomy and limited to the irradiated field occurring in a time frame consistent with sequelae of radiation therapy.

Clinical Aspects

▶ **Typical presentation**
Often asymptomatic • Symptoms may otherwise include cough, subfebrile temperatures, dyspnea with restrictive ventilation defect, elevated erythrocyte sedimentation rate, and leukocytosis.

▶ **Therapeutic options**
Steroids.

▶ **Course and prognosis**
Good.

▶ **What does the clinician want to know?**
Confirmation of the tentative diagnosis. • Follow-up examination in symptomatic patients.

Differential Diagnosis

Superinfection	– Not limited to the irradiated field
	– Clinical aspects
	– Course under therapy
Recurrent tumor	– Volume increase
	– New focal lesions
	– Peritumoral lymphangitis (can be difficult to distinguish; clinical course is important)

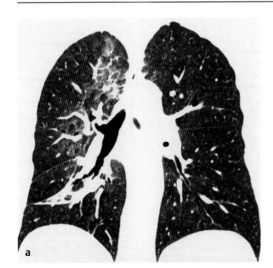

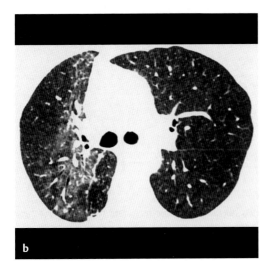

Fig. 13.4 Radiation pneumonitis in a 68-year-old man with bronchial carcinoma in the right lung. CT shows relatively sharply demarcated bandlike ground-glass opacity extending from anterior to posterior. The opacity includes the hilar region and does not respect anatomic boundaries.

Selected References

Choi YW et al. Effects of radiation therapy on the lung: radiologic appearances and differential diagnosis. Radiographics 2004; 24: 985–997

Libshitz HI. Radiation changes in the lung. Semin Roentgenol 1993; 28: 303–320

Definition

▶ **Epidemiology**
Direct sequela of lung transplantation, occurring in about 50% of cases.
▶ **Etiology, pathophysiology, pathogenesis**
Occurs within 48 hours of transplantation • Sequela of increased capillary permeability because of ischemia, impaired lymph drainage, and surfactant deficiency • Leads to interstitial and alveolar edema.

Imaging Signs

▶ **Modality of choice**
Radiographs • CT is not indicated as primary modality.
▶ **Radiographic and CT findings**
Changes due to edema include: Increased reticular shadowing • Bronchial wall thickening • Ground-glass opacity.
▶ **Pathognomonic findings**
Findings are nonspecific and are distinguishable from acute rejection or infection only by the time of their occurrence and their clinical course (see below).

Clinical Aspects

▶ **Typical presentation**
Hypoxemia.
▶ **Therapeutic options**
Oxygen administration • Avoid excessive hydration.
▶ **Course and prognosis**
Resolves within a week • Persistent or progressive findings suggest complications (acute transplant failure, rejection, infection).
▶ **What does the clinician want to know?**
Detection, localization, and extent of findings • Exclude pulmonary venous obstruction.

Differential Diagnosis

Early transplant failure	– Radiographically indistinguishable
	– Progressive hypoxia
Acute rejection	– Manifests later, with a different course: new or progressive shadows 5–6 days after lung transplantation
	– Fever
	– Dyspnea
	– Hypoxia
	– Diagnosis by biopsy
Infection	– Manifests later, with a different course
	– Focal consolidations and/or ground-glass opacities

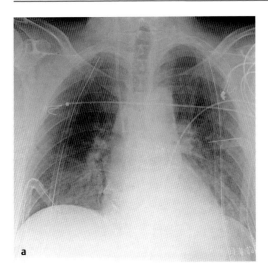

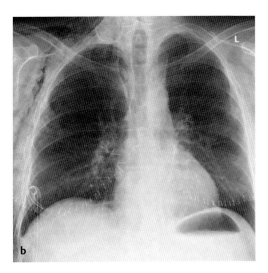

Fig. 13.5 Status post double lung transplantation in a 47-year-old man. The first plain chest radiograph (**a**) (postoperative day 2) shows a prominent ground-glass opacity in the lower lung fields and thickening of the bronchovascular bundles in the perihilar region indicative of fluid retention. By day 5 (**b**), the findings had largely resolved.

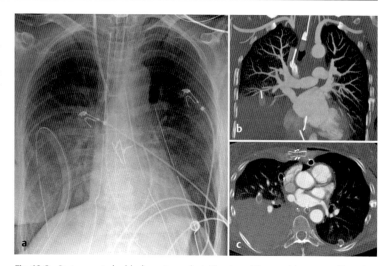

Fig. 13.6 Status post double lung transplantation in a 53-year-old woman. The plain chest radiograph (**a**) shows poorly delineated vascular structures, interstitial structures, and slight opacification with an apicobasal gradient on the left and in the right upper lung field. These findings are consistent with reperfusion edema. The right lower lung field is homogeneously dense. As this finding persisted during the further course of the condition, it could not be attributed to a reimplantation effect. Pneumonia was excluded. The subsequent CT scan (**b, c**) demonstrates complete occlusion of the veins of the right lower lobe consistent with early complications.

Selected References

Krishnam MS et al. Postoperative complications of lung transplantation: Radiologic findings along a time continuum. Radiographics 2007; 27: 957–974

Marom EM et al. Reperfusion edema after lung transplantation: Effect of daclizumab. Radiology 2001; 221: 508–514

Definition

Bronchiolitis obliterans syndrome involves worsening of pulmonary function due to peripheral airway obstruction (FEV_1 drops below 80% of the initial value) • Bronchiolitis obliterans (if histologically confirmed).

▶ **Epidemiology**
Long-term complication • Occurs in 50–70% of lung transplant recipients, and in 2–10% of patients receiving autologous peripheral blood stem cell transplants.

▶ **Etiology, pathophysiology, pathogenesis**
Multifocal fibroproliferative obstruction of the small airways • Changes are irreversible.

Imaging Signs

▶ **Modality of choice**
CT on inspiration and expiration.

▶ **Radiographic findings**
Usually there are no significant findings • At most there will be signs of hyperinflation.

▶ **CT findings**
Findings include regional differences in the density of the pulmonary parenchyma (mosaic pattern) that increase or only become visible on the expiration scan • Note that in extensive bronchiolitis obliterans there may not be a recognizable difference in density between the inspiration and expiration scans.

▶ **Pathognomonic findings**
See "CT findings."

Clinical Aspects

▶ **Typical presentation**
Signs of airway obstruction • FEV_1 drops below the initial value.

▶ **Therapeutic options**
Immunosuppression to avoid acute rejection • Ciclosporin or tacrolimus (there is no curative therapy).

▶ **Course and prognosis**
Variable • Mortality is 25–55%.

▶ **What does the clinician want to know?**
Confirmation of the tentative diagnosis • Exclude other complications.

Fig. 13.7 Bronchiolitis obliterans syndrome 14 months after lung transplantation (m, 53 y). The plain chest radiograph (**a**) shows a reticular pattern with peribronchial cutting and a loss of volume. The CT in inspiration (**b**) shows mild peripheral bronchiectasis (not shown) and a reticular pattern. The correspondent slice (**c**) shows air trapping as a sign for peribronchiolitic obstruction.

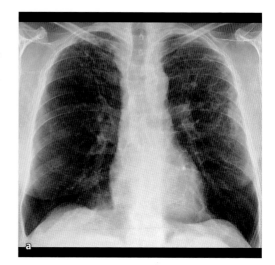

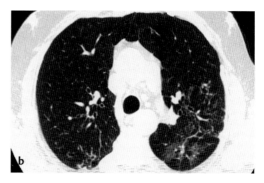

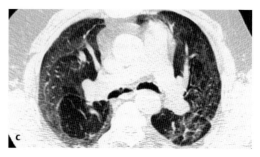

Differential Diagnosis

Mosaic pattern	– Regional ground-glass infiltrates, no air trapping
	– Mosaic perfusion in pulmonary embolism, no air trapping
	– Mosaic pattern due to irregular edema in preexisting pulmonary disease (chronic obstructive pulmonary disease, fibrosis), no air trapping

Tips and Pitfalls

False-negative findings may occur in the absence of a mosaic pattern ● In such cases correct expiration is recognizable only by compression or collapse of the central airways (trachea, main bronchi).

Selected References

Bankier AA et al. Bronchiolitis obliterans syndrome in heart-lung transplant recipients: diagnosis with expiratory CT. Radiology 2001; 218: 533–539

Boehler A, Estenne M. Obliterative bronchiolitis after lung transplantation. Curr Opin Pulm Med 2000; 6: 133–139

Estenne M et al. Bronchiolitis obliterans syndrome 2001: an update of the diagnostic criteria. J Heart Lung Transplant 2002; 21: 297–310

Definition

▶ **Epidemiology**
Noninfectious early complication in the neutropenic phase following bone marrow or peripheral blood stem cell transplantation.

▶ **Etiology, pathophysiology, pathogenesis**
Increased capillary permeability leads to edema (capillary leak syndrome) • This is the most common cause of pulmonary findings in the first 30 days aside from cardiac pathology or excessive hydration • Infections in this phase account for no more than 20% of cases • Later (30–180 days postoperatively) pneumonia is common (idiopathic pulmonary syndrome is the most important entity to consider in a differential diagnosis).

Imaging Signs

▶ **Modality of choice**
Radiographs • CT where clinical findings strongly suggest pulmonary pathology despite normal radiographs.

▶ **Radiographic findings**
Normal findings to bilateral alveolar opacities • Redistribution • Pleural effusion.

▶ **CT findings**
Bilateral ground-glass opacification with or without consolidations in the perihilar and peribronchial regions • Thickened interlobar septa.

▶ **Pathognomonic findings**
None (radiographic findings are nonspecific).

Clinical Aspects

▶ **Typical presentation**
Neutropenic phase (first 30 days) fever, skin changes as in graft-versus-host disease, hypoxemia.

▶ **Therapeutic options**
Supportive treatment.

▶ **Course and prognosis**
Good • Resolves spontaneously.

▶ **What does the clinician want to know?**
Adjunct to clinical diagnostic workup • Monitoring efficiency of treatment.

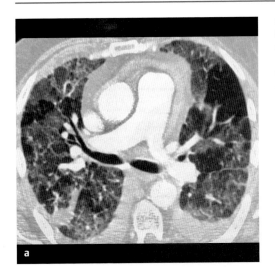

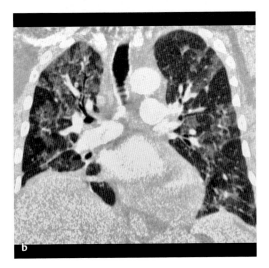

Fig. 13.8 Engraftment syndrome in a 65-year-old man with increasing respiratory insufficiency after peripheral blood stem cell transplantation 10 days previously. CT shows broad areas of ground-glass opacification distributed over both lungs in a mosaic pattern. Bilateral pleural and pericardial effusion, more pronounced on the right.

Differential Diagnosis

Edema	– Edema (from capillary leak, cardiac pathology, or excessive hydration) is the most common cause of pulmonary findings in the first 30 days
Parenchymal bleeding	– Severe complication, typically occurring as neutropenia subsides about 1 month after peripheral blood stem cell transplantation
Drug-induced lung disease	– Variably manifests itself as diffuse alveolar damage, nonspecific interstitial pneumonitis, etc. – Morphologically indistinguishable
Idiopathic pneumonia syndrome	– Diffuse lung damage without a detectable infection – Diagnosis of exclusion
Pneumonia	– Radiographic morphology varies; findings may be negative in the neutropenic phase – Bacteria, fungi, viruses (in order of decreasing importance)

Tips and Pitfalls

Misinterpretation of abnormal pulmonary findings.

Selected References

Evans A et al. Imaging in hematopoetic stem cell transplantation. Clin Radiol 2003; 58: 201–214

Khurshid I, Anderson LC. Non-infectious pulmonary complications after bone marrow transplantation. Postgrad Med J 2002; 78: 257–262

Wah TM et al. Pulmonary complications following bone marrow transplantation. Br J Radiol 2003; 76: 373–379

Definition

Central venous catheters are increasingly placed in patients in intensive care to monitor cardiovascular parameters such as central venous pressure and for medical treatment, especially for administration of locally irritating substances such as chemotherapy agents • Regardless of the specific catheter design, its tip invariably lies in the superior vena cava.

▶ **Types**
Several different types are used depending on the specific application:
  – *Simple central venous catheter:* The internal jugular vein or subclavian vein is catheterized using the Seldinger technique • These catheters are intended for short-term use perioperatively or in the intensive care unit (maximum of 14 days due to risk of infection) • The catheter provides up to five ports for infusion of incompatible drugs.
  – *Tunneled Hickman or Broviak catheter:* Central venous catheter with a long subcutaneous course and a Dacron cuff, which is implanted in a surgical or interventional procedure • Reduced risk of infection • Applications include at-risk patients, such as those receiving a bone marrow transplant; catheter residence time is necessarily longer.
  – *Dialysis catheter (Shaldon or Demers):* Double-channel or wide-channel catheter designed for high rates (up to 400 mL/min) and placed using the Seldinger technique • Used in dialysis.
  – *Peripherally inserted central venous catheter:* Central venous catheter with a relatively narrow lumen inserted through a peripheral brachial or basilic vein • Low rate of infection and minimal complications • Used for prolonged catheter residence (up to 6 months).
  – *Port catheter:* Complete system that can be placed subcutaneously, consisting of a chamber whose silicone membrane face can be repeatedly punctured, coupled to a central venous catheter • Ensures minimal complications with a good cosmetic result • Used for ambulant central venous therapy and designed for prolonged catheter residence up to several years.
  – *Pulmonary artery catheter (Swan–Ganz catheter):* This is placed using the Seldinger technique like a simple central venous catheter but then advanced through the right heart into the lower pulmonary artery • Used for monitoring cardiovascular parameters.

Imaging Signs

▶ **Modality of choice**
Radiographs to verify proper function and placement and to exclude complications; CT is used where indicated.

▶ **Radiographic findings**
Normal catheter position is in the vena cava or at the level of the cavoatrial junction • The tip of the catheter should be projected about 3 cm below the carina • Improper positioning: A catheter lying in the subclavian or brachiocephalic vein has not been advanced far enough, entailing a risk of thrombosis due to irritation

of the venous wall • A catheter lying within the atrium has been advanced too far, entailing a risk of arrhythmia due to mechanical irritation or myocardial perforation from a rigid catheter • The catheter may also be deflected or advanced into another vein (jugular, subclavian, azygos, or a thoracic or pericardiacophrenic vein) • Improper positioning in an artery may result from advancing the catheter into the common carotid or subclavian artery • Catheters may also be improperly positioned in extravascular locations such as the pleural space.

Clinical Aspects
....

▶ **Typical presentation**
Asymptomatic where properly positioned • Symptomatic complications may result from improper positioning: Extravascular position precludes injection and/or aspiration • Hematoma • Pneumothorax • Hydrothorax • Nerve injury • Sepsis • Thrombosis • Catheter fracture • Disconnection of a catheter from its port chamber.

▶ **Therapeutic options**
Improper positioning and/or complications are corrected by either repositioning the catheter or removing it and reinserting it.

▶ **What does the clinician want to know?**
Verify correct position • Where indicated, evaluate possible improper positioning or complication (such as catheter thrombosis).

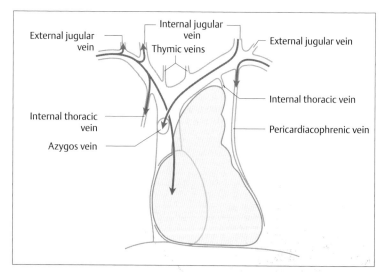

Fig. 13.9 Most common malpositions of a central venous catheter inserted through the subclavian or jugular vein.

Tips and Pitfalls

An atypical course of a catheter may be misinterpreted as improper positioning in the presence of a vascular anomaly such as a left or double superior vena cava.

Selected References

Gebauer B, Beck A, Wagner HJ. [Zentralvenöse Katheter: Diagnostik von Komplikationen und therapeutische Optionen.] Radiologie up2date 2008; 8: 135–152 [In German]

Schuster M et al. The carina as a landmark in central venous catheter placement. Br J Anaesth 2000; 85: 192–194

Vesely TM. Central venous catheter tip position: a continuing controversy. J Vasc Interv Radiol 2003; 14: 527–534

Definition

Implanted in patients with conduction disorders.

▶ **Types**
The pacemaker unit is placed subcutaneously on the pectoralis muscle, less often in the anterior abdominal wall • The pacing lead or leads course subcutaneously to a major vein of the thoracic inlet and are advanced from there to the heart.

– *Single-chamber pacemaker:* One pacing lead that terminates in the atrium (AAI) or ventricle (VVI) • Senses atrial and ventricular stimuli, and generates pulses when necessary • VVI pacing is indicated in chronic atrial fibrillation with bradycardiac conduction, AAI pacing in sick sinus syndrome with absent stimulation but an intact conduction system.

– *Dual-chamber pacemaker:* Most often this is a DDD pacemaker • It has an atrial and a ventricular lead for detecting stimuli and transmitting pacing pulses • By triggering excitation between the atrium and ventricle, this stimulation best approximates physiologic conduction • DDD pacemakers are used especially in an AV conduction block.

– *Biventricular (three-chamber) pacemakers:* In addition to the atrial and ventricular leads, a third lead is advanced via the coronary sinus as far as the posterolateral wall of the left ventricle • Additional left ventricular stimulation can achieve resynchronization in patients with left bundle branch block or symptomatic limited ventricular function (this prevents oscillating current).

– *Epicardial pacing leads:* Temporary cardiac stimulators after heart surgery • Intraoperative transcutaneous epicardial implantation • Only suitable for short-term use.

– *Cardioverter-defibrillators:* Combined pacemaker and defibrillator in recurrent ventricular tachycardia • Leads are placed as with a dual-chamber pacemaker but using thicker, stranded conductors.

Imaging Signs

▶ **Modality of choice**
Chest radiograph to verify position and exclude complications.

▶ **Radiographic findings**
Normal lead position: Atrial lead hangs on the atrial appendage • Ventricular lead hangs on the apex of the right ventricle • The left ventricular lead (three-chamber pacemaker) extends into the coronary sinus (toward the right shoulder on the posteroanterior film, posteriorly on the lateral film).

Clinical Aspects

▶ **What does the clinician want to know?**
Verify position of the leads after implantation • Proper function is confirmed electrophysiologically.

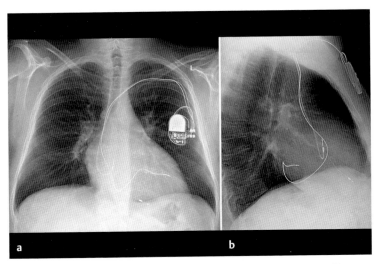

Fig. 13.10 Three-chamber pacemaker. Normal lead position with the atrial lead hanging on the right atrium and the ventricular lying on the right ventricle. The additional left ventricular lead passes around the base of the heart in the coronary sinus and terminates posteriorly, projected on the posterior wall.

Tips and Pitfalls

Complications such as a lead perforation or fracture are easily missed ● A lead with a nonradiodense segment can be misinterpreted as a fractured lead.

Selected References

Bauersfeld UK et al. Malposition of transvenous pacing lead in the left ventricle: radiographic findings. AJR Am J Roentgenol 1994; 162: 290–292

Daly BD et al. Nonthoracotomy lead implantable cardioverter defibrillators: normal radiographic appearance. AJR Am J Roentgenol 1993; 161: 749–752

Kaul TK, Bain WH. Radiographic appearances of implanted transvenous endocardial pacing electrodes. Chest 1977; 72: 323–326

Definition

▶ **Epidemiology**
Deposition of calcium salts in normal pulmonary parenchyma in metabolic disorders with hypercalcemia (primary or secondary hyperparathyroidism).

▶ **Etiology, pathophysiology, pathogenesis**
Hypercalcemia from various causes (such as primary or secondary hyperparathyroidism, terminal renal insufficiency, hypervitaminosis D, milk-alkali syndrome) ● Alkali environment is a predisposing factor ● Calcium deposits occur primarily in the alveolar septa and less often in the walls of arterioles and bronchioles.

Imaging Signs

▶ **Modality of choice**
CT.

▶ **Radiographic findings**
Nonspecific and not sensitive ● Only severe cases show diffuse ill-defined opacities.

▶ **CT findings**
Amorphous centrilobular "mulberry" densities of varying degree (from ground-glass to consolidating to isodense with calcification; measurements often fail to verify calcifications) with variable distribution (regionally localized or generalized) ● There may be associated vascular calcifications in the chest wall.

▶ **Pathognomonic findings**
See "CT findings" ● Vascular calcifications in addition to the underlying disorder can be diagnostic.

Clinical Aspects

▶ **Typical presentation**
Depending on severity, patients may be asymptomatic or may exhibit restricted lung function and reduced diffusion capacity.

▶ **Therapeutic options**
Management of the metabolic disorder or underlying disorder.

▶ **Course and prognosis**
Reversible in the early stages ● Chronic disease leads to fibrosis ● Prognosis depends on the underlying disorder.

▶ **What does the clinician want to know?**
Exclude parenchymal lesions of infectious, inflammatory, and immunologic etiology.

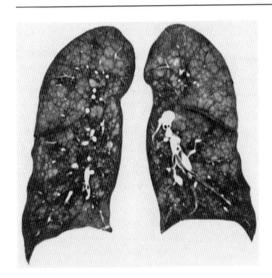

Fig. 13.11 Pulmonary parenchymal calcifications in secondary hyperparathyroidism in a 45-year-old man with terminal renal insufficiency. CT shows extensive cloudy, relatively sharply demarcated and relatively dense opacifications consistent with parenchymal calcifications. Density measurements are not conclusive as the measured volumes invariably include aerated alveoli in addition to parenchymal calcifications.

Differential Diagnosis

Alveolar microlithiasis
– Disseminated fine calcifications measuring only 1 mm, more pronounced in the basal segments
– Paraseptal emphysema
– No history

Tips and Pitfalls

Can be misinterpreted as edema or atypical pneumonia.

Selected References

Hartman TE et al. Metastatic pulmonary calcification in patients with hypercalcemia: findings on chest radiographs and CT scans. AJR Am J Roentgenol 1994; 162: 799–802

Lingam RK et al. Metastatic pulmonary calcification in renal failure: a new HRCT pattern. Br J Radiol 2002; 75: 74–77

Page locators in *italics* indicate
illustrations.